Congregate Housing for the Elderly: Theoretical, Policy, and Programmatic Perspectives

Congregate Housing for the Elderly: Theoretical, Policy, and Programmatic Perspectives

Lenard W. Kaye
Abraham Monk
Editors

The Haworth Press, Inc.
New York • London • Sydney

Congregate Housing for the Elderly: Theoretical, Policy, and Programmatic Perspectives has also been published as *Journal of Housing for the Elderly*, Volume 9, Numbers 1/2 1991.

The Haworth Press, Inc., 10 Alice Street, Binghamton, NY 13904-1580
EUROSPAN/Haworth, 3 Henrietta Street, London WC2E 8LU England
ASTAM/Haworth, 162-168 Parramatta Road, Stanmore, Sydney, N.S.W. 2048 Australia

Library of Congress Cataloging-in-Publication Data

Congregate housing for the elderly: theoretical, policy and programmatic perspectives/Lenard W. Kaye, Abraham Monk, editors.
    p. cm.
    ISBN 1-56024-227-2 (H: alk. paper). —ISBN 1-56024-228-0 (S: alk. paper)
    1. Aged—Housing—United States. 2. Congregate housing—United States. I. Kaye, Lenard W. II. Monk, Abraham.
HD7287.92.U54C674 1992
363.5'946'0973—dc20
                                     91-33398
                                            CIP

Congregate Housing for the Elderly: Theoretical, Policy, and Programmatic Perspectives

CONTENTS

III. PROGRAMMATIC PERSPECTIVES

IV. FUTURE PERSPECTIVES

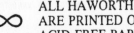

ALL HAWORTH BOOKS & JOURNALS
ARE PRINTED ON CERTIFIED
ACID-FREE PAPER

ABOUT THE EDITORS

Lenard W. Kaye, DSW, is Professor and Associate Dean at the Bryn Mawr College Graduate School of Social Work and Social Research. Formerly, he was Associate Director of the Brookdale Institute on Aging and Adult Human Development and faculty member at Columbia University School of Social Work. The co-author of several books, including *Resolving Grievances in the Nursing Home* and *Men as Caregivers to the Elderly: Understanding and Aiding Unrecognized Family Support*, Dr. Kaye has also published more than fifty journal articles and book chapters on issues in nursing home advocacy, home health care, elder caregiving, retirement lifestyles, and long-term care. His forthcoming book is titled *Geriatric Case Practice in Home Health Care*. He has recently completed research on the part-time work experiences of lower-income elderly funded in part by the Families USA Foundation and on marketing techniques in health and social services for the elderly supported by a grant from the AARP Andrus Foundation. His current research, funded by the AARP Andrus Foundation, addresses the development of "best-practice" models for structuring self help support groups for older women. Dr. Kaye, a Fellow of the Gerontological Society of America, is a member of the editorial boards of the *Journal of Gerontological Social Work* and *Research on Social Work Practice*.

Abraham Monk, PhD, is Professor of Social Work and Gerontology at the Columbia University School of Social Work in New York City and Director of the Institute on Aging at Columbia University. He also served as Associate Director of the Long Term Care Gerontology Center of Columbia University's Faculty of Medicine. Dr. Monk has conducted extensive research on intergenerational relations, housing and sheltered environments, long term care, pre-retirement preparation and post-retirement adjustment, and policy formation concerning families of the aged. He has recently conducted a study of home care services in six countries, with a grant from the USDHHS-Administration on Aging. Prior to his affiliation with Columbia University, he was Professor of Social Work at the State University of New York in Buffalo and Director of its Multidisciplinary Center on Aging.

Dr. Monk is the author of over 100 publications in refereed scholarly and professional journals, as well as chapters in several books in the fields of aging, social planning, and evaluative research. The author and editor of four books, the revised, second edition of his *Handbook of Gerontological Services* was released in Spring 1990. He is the editor of a series of books titled the *Columbia Series of Social Gerontology and Aging*, launched in 1983 by Columbia University Press.

Dr. Monk is a Fellow of the American Gerontological Society and served as its Vice President. He has received numerous awards including a Fulbright Senior Scholarship and has served as consultant to many international, national, governmental, and voluntary service organizations in the field of aging.

Preface

In the early decades of this century, old people and their families had to fend for themselves and for each other. When that was no longer possible, there were no available alternative solutions to the disgrace of "going to the poor farm" or almshouse. During the century's mid-decades, some attempts were made to develop publicly and privately supported programs to change the unhappy circumstances of the poor and near poor elderly wherever they lived. Then in 1963 President Kennedy, in a message to the Congress, set forth the basic concept of what later was to be incorporated into national programs of congregate housing. In that message he said:

> For the great majority of the Nation's older people the years of retirement should be years of activity and self-reliance. A substantial minority, however, while still relatively independent, require modest assistance in one or more aspects of their daily living. Many have become frail physically and may need help in preparing meals, caring for living quarters, and sometimes limited nursing.

> This group does not require care in restorative nursing homes or in terminal custodial facilities. They can generally walk without assistance, eat in a dining room, and come and go in the community with considerable independence. They want to have privacy but also community life and activity within the limits of their capacity. They do not wish to be shunted to an institution, but often they have used up their resources; and family and friends are not available for support. What they do need most is a facility with housekeeping assistance, central food service, and minor nursing from time to time. The provision of such facilities would defer for many years the much more expensive type of nursing home or hospital care which would otherwise be required.[1]

President Kennedy went on to recommend that housing programs be enacted that would incorporate the services he had outlined.

This action was finally taken in 1970 when the Congress passed legislation that included funds for the construction of congregate housing for the elderly. In 1974, the Congress reaffirmed the congregate housing program

ix

and included authorization for inclusion of space for central kitchen and dining rooms, equipment, and such operating expenses as electricity, heat, and maintenance. Four years later in 1978, the Congress enacted legislation authorizing subsidies to provide services for impaired elderly residents of congregate housing.

These events constituted the foundation for the large number of approaches to the congregate housing concept. Whatever the approach, the broad goal of congregate housing for the elderly is to provide a physical and social environment that will extend the time span during which older people can live independently in comfort and safety, and with an enduring interest in life. More specifically, it makes available to older people a choice of living arrangements between fully independent facilities and institutional facilities and hence bridges a long existing gap in the shelter continuum. It also provides environments of housing and services specially designed to accommodate declining functional capacities associated with growing older. Finally, and perhaps most importantly, it offers a stimulating environment that provides opportunities for growth, which helps to prevent or at least slows the onset of preventable mental and physical changes often associated with old age.

Drs. Kaye and Monk have put together an excellent set of readings that promise not only to update the state of the art of congregate housing experiences and issues, but to raise the level of societal awareness of this important housing alternative. This is an articulate and timely work that will inform the important actors in this field — legislators, policy makers, lending institutions, researchers, developers and designers, providers, advocates and most importantly the elderly themselves — regarding the present and future impact this housing and living arrangement alternative has had and will have in the years ahead.

Leon A. Pastalan

NOTE

1. U.S. House of Representatives. President Kennedy's message on aid to elderly citizens, House Document 72. The House, Washington, DC, February 21, 1963.

Introduction

The availability of various types of noninstitutional housing for the elderly has grown at a lively pace in recent years. Shared housing, life care, continuing care retirement communities, "granny flats," NORCs (Naturally Occurring Retirement Communities), and accessory apartments are rapidly becoming common parlance among gerontological researchers and practitioners. One category of planned older adult housing of relatively recent popularity has been alternately labeled enriched, congregate, or service-assisted housing. These intermediate, community-based, supportive environments for the elderly are quickly assuming a prominent position in the gerontological services continuum as well.

In part fueled by the widespread popularity of a variety of program alternatives to institutionalization, congregate housing is now considered a desirable service option for those elderly and disabled who are now or anticipate in the near future experiencing limited degrees of functional impairment. While most older people may continue to prefer to live on their own in free-standing housing, in a recent national survey of 1,500 adults age 55 and older sponsored by the American Association of Retired Persons (AARP), almost one in three said they would consider moving into a congregate housing facility (1990). This same AARP survey found that seven percent of the elderly respondents had already moved into a congregate apartment house or were seriously considering doing so.

Amidst the popularity of congregate housing, however, has emerged the reality of the "aging-in" or "aging-in-place" phenomenon. The same AARP study cited above found that a majority of older people would like to age in their habitual homes and consequently expect to need assistance with household maintenance responsibilities in order to remain independent. In similar fashion, the aging-in process is already playing itself out among elders residing in congregate facilities such as those funded through the Section 202 Housing Program for the Elderly. A study conducted by the Housing Research and Development Program at the University of Illinois at Urbana-Champaign reports that the average age of residents living in this type of housing rose from 72 years in 1983 to 75 years in 1988 (American Association of Retired Persons, 1989-90).

The implications of progressive aging among residents of congregate housing developments rather than serving to cool interest in this interventive strategy, are likely to represent a sobering reality which will further challenge policymakers, planners and administrators of congregate housing. The 1990s promise to bring continued efforts at conceptualizing and operationalizing creative forms of noninstitutional service-assisted housing for older adults. In support of those efforts and with the intent of providing a view to the future, this special collection of original articles represents some of the most recent research and thinking on a variety of important topics pertaining to congregate housing in the areas of theory, policy, and program development.

A variety of perspectives have been deliberately sought from authorities engaged in different aspects of elder housing and environmental analysis. Theoreticians, policy analysts, researchers, administrators, planners and designers, and legislative and consumer advocates are all represented.

Monk and Kaye commence with a review of the current status of congregate housing for the elderly and the relationship between aging and the housing environment. Golant then considers from a theoretical perspective the difficult challenge of successfully matching housing and residents. Kingsley and Struyk proceed to paint a scenario of the future of congregate housing in the context of the unfolding course of general housing policy in the United States. The reader is then presented with the findings of a recent state-wide survey reported by Granger and Kaye that sought to gauge the relative demand and need for congregate-type housing for older adults in one state—Pennsylvania. Heumann subsequently presents just completed research findings that succeed in documenting the relative changes in the cost of elder care in congregate versus long-term care facilities over a five year period, 1985 to 1990. The policy discussion concludes with a revealing personal perspective from two experienced legislative and consumer advocates, Redfoot and Sloan, concerning the process of federal decision-making on issues in congregate housing.

Selected programmatic aspects of congregate housing are then brought to the fore. Kaye and Monk report on a case study analysis of the integrity of social relationships among elder congregate housing residents in a New York City facility. Hunt then proceeds to discuss a series of pertinent issues in designing supportive environments for older adults. Warach offers a richly detailed history of one agency's experience in promoting a variety of initiatives in service-assisted housing for older people. Fairchild, Higgins, and Folts close this section by tracing the evolution of proprietary involvement in the field of supportive housing.

Finally, Lawton outlines a compelling scenario of the future, offering his view of the critical questions and challenges that remain to be confronted in the years ahead in elder housing.

We hope this set of articles both answers questions and raises issues for those engaged in shaping the future of congregate housing. If it does, it will have succeeded in its purpose.

Lenard W. Kaye
Abraham Monk
Editors

REFERENCES

American Association of Retired Persons. (December/January 1989-90). "Congressional Study Finds That Regulations Reduce Effectiveness of Section 202 Program." *AARP Housing Report*, p. 3.

American Association of Retired Persons. (Spring 1990). "AARP's 1990 Housing Survey Shows More Older People Want to Age in Place." *AARP Housing Report*, p. 1.

Congregate Housing for the Elderly: Its Need, Function and Perspectives

Abraham Monk
Lenard W. Kaye

INTRODUCTION

The relationship between old age and the housing environment continues to intrigue policy makers, social planners and service providers. It is also a major concern for those seniors who begin experiencing physical and cognitive frailties and can no longer manage adequately in their homes. Even in the absence of such functional limitations, many "well" aged find that their homes have ceased to meet their needs: they may be overhoused once loved ones depart or die; they may feel lonely and cut off from other people; they may feel threatened in a neighborhood that has become unsafe; and they may not be able to bear the maintenance costs. In sum, it may not be feasible or advisable for them to continue their habitual style of independent living, but, on the other hand, they are still far from needing placement in a nursing home type of facility.

For years, policy makers and social planners accepted the rather simplistic dichotomy between independent living and long term care institutionalization. Heumann and Brody (1982) pointed out that the dichotomy in question was perpetuated by two separate courses of action in public policy. The first took place immediately after World War II and it was aimed at putting a roof over the head of millions of low income persons. It was a "brick and mortar only" policy because it did not consider attaching any form of services to the newly built housing stock. The second occurred a couple of decades later when Congress amended the Social

Abraham Monk, PhD, is Professor of Social Work at the Columbia University School of Social Work in New York City. Lenard W. Kaye, DSW, is Professor and Associate Dean at the Bryn Mawr College Graduate School of Social Work and Social Research in Bryn Mawr, PA.

5

Security Act and introduced Title XIX, or Medicaid, as a main source of financing the health and maintenance care of low income frail elderly in nursing homes. Heumann and Brody added that this separation between housing and health service still conspired against a solution to the growing demand for long term care. They consequently argued for a convergence whereby housing programs will venture beyond the mere design of physical structures into the service needs of residents and, conversely, health care programs for the aged will constitute an inseparable component of their housing environment. This convergence has gradually evolved in the form of a series of alternative forms of residence, but their creation took place more by trial and error than by calculated design.

The resulting intermediate housing models constitute a *de facto* continuum that is responsive to the gradually declining levels of physical, functional and mental ability as the elderly grow older. They also take into account concurrent changes in the familial and social circumstances of this population. At least three sets of factors are seen as having created this diversity of housing models for the aged.

First are the well-known realities of a changing demographic profile in the United States. Longer life expectancy and increased likelihood of functional impairment associated with age have each led to an increasing number of old people who are at risk of needing specialized housing and housing-related supports at some point in their lives (Struyk and Soldo, 1980; U.S. Department of Housing and Urban Development, 1983).

Second are the economic realities. The *Report of the Mini-White House Conference on Housing for the Elderly* (1981) pointed out that 20% or 14.8 million of the nation's households are now headed by someone 65 years or older, and that their median income was nearly 60% below that of the population as a whole. Furthermore, despite the fact that nearly three-quarters of the elderly were homeowners, and most (84%) have paid their mortgages, 30% of the elderly live in substandard and deteriorating housing stock, without central heat or complete plumbing and kitchen facilities. Nearly 60% of the aged home-owners live in homes they purchased before 1939. The elderly, in addition, are known to spend larger proportions of their income than others for food, health care, and, in particular, housing, for which individuals over the age of 75 pay almost half of their income (U.S. Congress, House Select Committee on Aging, 1988). The latter is the largest single budget item for retired couples. Furthermore, the housing occupied by nearly half of the elderly is more than 40 years old and thus both poorly insulated and subject to high maintenance costs.

The Urban Institute estimated that some 2.4 million persons aged 65 and above need appropriate shelter and services to remain outside of institutions (Department of Health and Human Services, 1981).

A third set of factors is largely of a social nature. Included here is the trend away from intergenerational living arrangements and the fact that older people move much less frequently than do those of working age. Only about 6% of those aged 65 and over move in any given year, which is only about one-quarter the rate for adults under the age of 65 (Lawton, 1980). The increasing and relentless losses experienced by the aged in their social and familial networks also impact on the quality and quantity of relationships in their housing environment, the symbolic and affective connotations attached to their home, their feelings of environmental security, and their access to services and resources. Several concurrent factors that also gravitate on the elderly housing market are: (1) Current and anticipated migratory patterns. The well aged wishing to migrate proceed to the sun belt, while frail elderly return north to their original home bases (Longino, 1979); (2) The close association between housing deficiencies and permanent poverty (Newman, 1985); (3) The excessive costs of upkeep, maintenance and local taxes for the 75% of the aged who are homeowners; (4) The reduction of rental housing by destruction, abandonment and conversions; and (5) The shrinking levels of governmental housing assistance for low and moderate income families.

It should be noted, however, that despite the availability of many senior housing options, the majority of older people want to remain in their homes and familiar communities. It is simply not true that people just pack and move when they retire. Studies and census data refute this "mobility myth." Only 30% of older persons move sometime after they reach 65 years of age; only 3% buy or rent new homes; and only 4% move out of the state in which they lived after age 65 (Baldwin, 1980). "Staying put" or "aging in place" is the prevailing trend.

The numerous models of intermediate housing have consequently responded to the needs of older persons who do not wish or cannot manage to live alone, or who no longer can handle the challenges of their home environment. Many of the models or alternatives have already been tested in practice, while others are still on the planning board or in an incipient stage of development. The former include domiciliary care homes, homes for the aged, foster care homes, life care or continuing care communities, and finally retirement communities, both of the intentional type and NORCs (Naturally Occurring Retirement Communities) and, of course, congregate housing.

CONGREGATE HOUSING
DEFINITION AND GOALS

Congregate housing is positioned between the more protective environments of skilled and intermediate care facilities and largely independent environments such as retirement communities, private homes, and apartments. Congregate housing has been defined as:

> a residential setting that is non-institutional, but adapted to meet the special needs of the elderly persons through good design of the physical environment and the provision of some supportive services. It offers the functionally impaired or socially deprived, but not ill elderly, residential accommodations to assist them in maintaining or returning to an independent or semi-independent lifestyle and prevent premature or unnecessary institutionalization as they grow older. (Cronin et al., 1983, p. 1)

There are many different conceptions as to what constitutes congregate housing. Professionals use different terms to describe it depending on the state, sponsor, and type of structure. Common terms are enriched housing, sheltered housing, and shared housing. Most facilities have separate apartments for each resident plus common shared areas for meals and recreation. Some have private bedrooms plus common shared areas such as the living and dining rooms and kitchen. Whatever term and design used, the intent of a congregate program is to provide services in a residential setting for resident persons who can no longer single-handedly manage the tasks of everyday living, in ordinary community housing. Residents must consequently have a degree of limitation that, in the absence of enriched or congregate housing, would preclude independent living, but that does not require continuous medical or nursing care nor fulltime personal care.

The report of the Council of State Housing Agencies and The National Association of State Units on Aging (1987) developed a more encompassing classification of congregate housing residents. It consists of these 6 categories:

a. The physically "well" but not wishing to live alone;
b. The physically "well" but who need to feel needed by others;
c. The physically "well" but in need of the emotional support that results from living with others;
d. The physically "capable" but in need of assistance to gain back a

relatively independent lifestyle (for example, a person who has been hospitalized or in a nursing home);

e. The physically "unwell" or handicapped and in need of formal or informal support;

f. Those suffering some mental incapacity but can do things slowly and independently with some support.

This diversity of potential residents implies the need for a concomitant wide range of potential packages of services, as well as the built-in administrative flexibility for attending to each individual's needs.

HISTORY

Public housing tenants are aging in their apartments, and an increasing number of public housing authorities are constantly faced with the frailty and dependence of that population. In fact, a 1977 estimate revealed that 45,000 elderly faced eviction from public housing because of physical impairment (Health and Social Service and Housing Congressional Hearing, 1977 in Donahue et al., 1977). Thompson observed that public policy provides resources to maintain "public housing buildings as they age, but none to maintain the residents as they age." (Thompson, in Chellis et al., 1982).

The aging of residents in public housing gave impetus to the congregate housing movement. However, congregate housing is also needed beyond the public housing community, as only 3 to 4% of the older population live in public housing. Most older people own their own homes (72%) and the rest either live in nursing homes (5%) or rent apartments, single room occupancies, or homeshare with relatives or nonrelatives (23%) (AARP Profile of Older Americans, 1985).

The congregate housing concept surfaced in 1963 as a specific recommendation made by President Kennedy to Congress. It advocated the creation of a housing program that would include a communal living facility and services for low-income, frail elderly. After a number of unsuccessful attempts to pass such legislation, Congress finally included construction funds for congregate housing in the 1970 Housing and Community Development Act. Legislative support was reaffirmed by Section 7 of the Housing and Community Development Act of 1974, but the language of the bill was rather restrictive, as it was primarily concerned with the provision of dining rooms, kitchens, and equipment rather than with funding for food or personnel. Housing authorities found it difficult to shoulder on their own the costs of food and related support services. It was not until four years later that Congress established the Congregate Housing Services Program (CHSP) as Title IV of the Housing and Community Development Amendment of 1978.

One of the reasons for the long delay in establishing a congregate housing program that included services was that the Department of Housing and Urban Development felt that it would impose an institutional identity on public housing. Prior to the 1970 legislation, all on-site services in public housing for the elderly had to be sponsored by local agencies who often encountered great difficulties when attempting to secure loans to finance such projects (Lawton, 1976).

FEDERAL AND STATE INITIATIVES

The Congregate Housing Services Program (CHSP) is administered by HUD with the collaboration of the Administration on Aging (AoA), the State Units on Aging, and Area Agencies on Aging. Under this federally funded program, public housing authorities and non-profit Section 202 funded projects could apply for additional funds to provide meals, other supportive services, and "allowable" administrative costs. Residents of the CHSP were expected to pay for all services on a sliding scale basis.

There were 62 such congregate programs operating nationwide. Thirty-two of them were located in public housing, and 30 in Section 202 projects. The typical contract period has been three years but many of these contracts have been extended. According to Nachison (1985a) costs were reimbursed on a unit of service basis and monitoring followed contractual administration, not grants management practice. The legislation authorized service funds for 20% of the eligible low income residents who meet Activities of Daily Living criteria. Waivers were available for additional funds if a project exceeded the 20% guideline. The purpose of these guidelines was to prevent "institutionalizing" the facility.

Participants of CHSP had to be 62 years and over or a nonelderly handicapped person. Two hot meals had to be served seven days a week and these had to meet the nutritional standards outlined in the 1965 Older Americans Act.

The federal CHSP program was upgraded in 1987 from a demonstration to a regular, permanent program. As of 1988, 9 states continued running congregate housing programs. Struyk (1989) observed that they remain small demonstrations rarely exceeding a few hundred beneficiaries. Almost simultaneously, many Section 202 and other federally-assisted housing projects have been integrating support services in a way that brought them very close to the prevailing definition of congregate housing. It must be borne in mind that nearly 3 million elderly live in federally-assisted housing and that they have been rapidly aging in place. Yet their projects were originally conceived for the well aged, with little or no consideration of their imminent supportive services needs.

Another federally funded program was jointly initiated by Farmers Home Administration (FmHA) and the Administration on Aging. This national demonstration program established ten congregate housing projects in rural communities scattered in different regions of the United States. A memorandum of understanding between AoA and FmHA outlined the specific funding mechanisms to support the pilot project.

EVALUATING THE CHSP PROGRAM

In 1986 Sherwood et al., released the results of an evaluation of the CHSP program, commissioned by the U.S. Department of Housing and Urban Development. The study concluded that the program has been effective in preventing unnecessary institutionalization and that it constitutes a cost effective alternative to institutional care. Sherwood's report also pointed out that HUD's initial requirement of 2 meals a day, seven days a week, turned food into the program's center piece. Meals thus constituted 54% of the program's costs and over two-thirds of the time spent in the provision of organized services. The study concluded, however, that there was no evidence for the need of such intense emphasis on meals and recommended that the requirement be eliminated. HUD accepted this recommendation and put it into effect a year later (U.S. Congress, House Select Committee on Aging, 1987).

Kaye et al., (1985) similarly conducted a study of all the 62 CHSP grantees funded by the U.S. Department of Housing and Human Development and targeted a sample of 10 sites for in-depth and on-site visits. Of these 10 sites, 6 were originally funded under Section 202 and 4 were public housing authorities. Five of the sites were located within the New York City Metropolitan area and 5 were scattered across the country.

Interviews were conducted and questionnaires were administered to program administrators, service workers and the elderly residing in these enriched housing programs.

Taken together, the congregate housing programs surveyed were rated positively by both the staff and residents. The programs were thought to be most effective in their ability to improve the nutrition of the participants, prolong independence, provide companionship, improve self-worth, develop a sense of community, and reduce isolation. It was felt that residents were able to live in their own apartments for a longer period of time than they would have been without these supports.

Residents were for the most part satisfied with both their living conditions and the program. The most frequently cited advantage of a site was the package of services it made available. This was followed by the increased opportunity for socialization and the reduction in the number of respondents who felt isolated.

While over two-thirds of the respondents reported having physical problems or disabilities, they also were found to have relatively high life satisfaction scores. The oldest respondents were those who indicated the highest scores on the life satisfaction index.

Residents used an average of 9 congregate housing services. Those that received the highest satisfaction scores were preventive medicine, transportation, personal care, housekeeping services and counseling. Less satisfaction was expressed with regard to educational classes, special programs for the handicapped/disabled, rehabilitation services, recreational activities, and the meals served in the dining hall.

Residents established good rapport and trust with staff and stated they would turn first to them in an emergency. Residents also claimed they relied on CHSP staff most often for cooking and household chores.

Not all of the evaluations were, however, positive. Program limitations most often cited were a lack of recreational activities and program inflexibility, especially as it related to the meals program.

In a study of 27 private congregate facilities conducted under the auspices of Urban Systems, Malozemoff and his associates found that these study sites also provided a mean of nine services, with 56% of the sites making available a medium to high level of service (1978). In those instances where the number of on-site services was low, managers had apparently made efforts to link residents to community services by providing transportation or arranging for community agencies to bring their services to the site. In addition, a sustained management commitment to extend services to residents often resulted in operating deficits at most sites.

Residents were free to choose among various services on a fee-for-service basis, or opt for one of a series of service packages, but some facilities had to charge a flat service fee to all residents.

Housekeeping was the most frequently requested service, with medical services ranking second. Meals constituted a very low priority. Only among a very old and relatively unhealthy segment of respondents was the meal service considered to be anything more than an amenity or convenience.

Malozemoff's study concluded by highlighting the problems that have arisen in the provision of services in congregate settings. The most significant were:

- The inflationary pressure on cost of services;
- The residents' preference for costly on-site services such as medical care;
- Lack of utilization of community resources by management to provide on-site services on either a voluntary or contractual basis which could have saved staff time and other costs;
- The ability of most residents to personalize and choose services, a fact that limits the economies of scale that could be derived from serving a large group more uniformly.

One solution proposed by the Urban Systems research team was the implementation of a prepayment service plan. They readily admitted, however, that this plan might detract from the residential atmosphere and encourage tenants to use services they might not really need.

WHO NEEDS CONGREGATE HOUSING?

It is estimated that there are currently 3 million elderly functionally eligible for congregate housing (Prosper, 1987). As a greater proportion of the population ages, consumer education will be required to cultivate a demand for the program. As observed by Pollack et al., the expression of interest does not necessarily predict that an older person will actually move in when congregate housing becomes available. The authors add that "many persons are unable to acknowledge their own need for service until their frailty has increased to the point that they need more than the program can offer" (1985, p. 7).

The major reasons their respondents had moved into congregate housing were, according to Malozemoff et al., 1978:

- loneliness (27% wanted to be in an environment where there would be more people they could be friends with).
- insecurity due to poor health status.
- availability of supportive services.

The type of service amenities available was more of a factor in an upper income bracket person's decision to move into congregate housing, while obtaining decent housing was the leading priority for lower income elderly.

On the whole, respondents stated that they saw themselves needing services in the future but not at the time of the survey. They viewed moving into congregate housing as a means of insuring services at a later date (Malozemoff et al., 1978).

Residents tend to choose congregate housing more because of housing needs than because of a perceived need for services, according to the Urban Systems study previously mentioned. Priorities guiding the choice of the congregate facility were location and accessibility. Lawton found that location was the most important criteria for entering congregate housing (Lawton, 1980). A 1969 study by Beckman, cited by Heumann, indicated that congregate living appeared more acceptable to those whose past lifestyles and occupations involved "human associations" — educators, social workers, etc. — rather than farmers, artists, and housewives without children (1976).

A study of 87 congregate housing applicants conducted by the Philadelphia Geriatric Center revealed that these urban elderly were seeking out congregate housing mostly because of fear of crime, poor conditions of current dwelling, loneliness and isolation, accessibility of services, and proximity to family, in this order of frequency (Lawton, 1976).

Conversely, applicants who had reservations about moving cited the following reasons:

• complaints about certain housing features, such as lack of tub;
• delays in completion of housing;
• reluctance to leave familiar surroundings;
• difficulty of moving; and decreasing physical strength.

It should be noted that respondents who ultimately moved into congregate housing had as many complaints as those who never made the move. However, reluctance to leave familiar surroundings turned out to be a much more powerful predictor of not moving than other reasons, since 70% of the non-movers gave this reason compared to 25% of the experimental group that actually moved to congregate housing (Brody, 1978).

THE EFFECTS OF CONGREGATE HOUSING ON RESIDENTS

There are conflicting findings regarding the effect of congregate housing on residents. Several studies (Monk et al., 1986; Kaye et al., 1985; Malozemoff et al., 1978) found no major change in tenants' activity patterns. They continued for the most part to visit friends, shop, and participate in outside clubs at the same pace as prior to the move. They did not begin to rely on on-site services until their health deteriorated to the point where they had to limit their travels outside the site. These studies also found that residents adapted fairly quickly to their new home and made friends fairly easily, although these social relations were in addition to and not a replacement for previous lifelong friendships.

In a study of residents of Brookdale Village, Monk et al., (1986) found that most perceive this congregate housing complex operated by the Jewish Association for Services for the Aged in New York City as a very good place to live, due mostly to the pleasant and aesthetical connotations of the physical environment. They also underscored its convenient proximity to health services and the conviviality of fellow tenants. Respondents also identified some of the least desirable aspects of living in that location. They mentioned, to this effect, the surrounding area's lack of safety and the lack of adequate public transportation. These shortcomings notwithstanding, the majority concurred that Brookdale Village was a pleasant and satisfying place to live.

Kaye et al. (1985) determined that respondents expressing lower satisfaction with the CHSP were also having greater difficulty in performing household tasks. The authors hypothesized that the lower satisfaction may be more a projection of diminishing ability for self care, than actual discontent with the services at hand. This finding may also reflect CHSP's inadequacy to attend to the needs of the more severely impaired.

Lawton (1976) examined the well-being of prospective tenants of similar health status who moved to either traditional or congregate housing. He found that the group which moved to traditional housing made gains in their "leisure patterns" and external involvement such as following the news, taking on new interests, or spending time outdoors, while those who moved to congregate housing improved in morale, social status, and housing satisfaction. They lost some ground, however, in the areas of leisure and external involvement. Lawton raised the question of whether these changes may be due as much, if not more, to each individual's rate of decline.

Cantor and Donovan (1982) found that the overall level of satisfaction with congregate housing was high. The noninstitutional character of a setting played an important role in the residents' perception of program success. Group needs were met and services were successfully tailored to individual requirements, with those needing more help receiving a greater number and intensity of services.

In a study of the FmHA demonstration, Cronin et al., observed that most tenants were satisfied with congregate living (1983). Although one in ten of the original pool of tenants left congregate housing voluntarily (that is, for reasons other than death, illness, or eviction), there has been no shortage of tenants to replace those who moved out. A high vacancy rate may be indicative of either an oversaturated market or an unsuccessful project.

CONCLUSION:
THE FUTURE OF CONGREGATE HOUSING

Congregate housing emerged nearly two decades ago as a product of the continuum of care concept and it soon received the endorsement of both policy makers and professionals in the field of aging. The first were attracted to its promise of a substantially lower cost-per-unit of service than the dreaded institutional alternative. Nachison pointed out, to this effect, that the CHSP succeeded in delivering noninstitutional support at half or even one-third of the cost of institutionalization (1985b). Professionals praised, in turn, the flexibility of congregate housing as a service model. Facilities, whether newly constructed or renovated, could therefore be adapted to constantly changing resident populations as well as varying service demands and community needs.

The CHSP program was the largest experiment ever undertaken by the federal government aimed at integrating housing environments and human services. It passed its initial fledgling demonstration stage and reached the level of statutory permanency. Parallel to it there were several other experiments that have been barely touched upon or not mentioned in this paper.

The introduction of congregate housing into the private, proprietary and the private, non-profit housing sectors was the pragmatic consequence of the "aging in" process taking place in all housing programs for the "well" elderly, rather than the result of a special ideological commitment. The increase in the number of frail residents brought housing managers to the realization that it is far more feasible to import community services into their premises, than force the wholesale relocation of their increasingly dependent tenants.

Time, however, does not seem in favor of the present, first generation of congregate housing programs. Their population, regardless of whether one deals with the public or the private sector, is aging across the board and just initiating the systematic provision of formal services to even a small number of residents may create, according to Prosper, the fear among the majority of the "well" residents that their housing facility is being converted into a nursing home (1987).

The concern that congregate housing may still become another type of institution stems from: (1) the inability to define an acceptable threshold of services. One may wonder whether there is an upper limit in the volume, variety, intensity and continuity of services that can be integrated without affecting the independent or semi-independent character of a given congregate housing project; (2) The potential negative effect of a package of systematic services upon the privacy of the residents; and (3) The effects of a facility's size on the community and residents' perception of its alleged noninstitutional character.

Concerning the first and second issue, even when congregate care programs tend to limit themselves to short term and intermittent nursing care, increasing numbers of residents are purchasing on their own more intensive and continuous home care services. The housing project may have its own policies but residents are free to do privately whatever they deem necessary to insure their continuity of residency. Of course, the import of private support services, individually paid and negotiated, may still impinge upon the very identity of the housing project.

The third concern poses a special planning dilemma. Developers are attuned to the economies of scale and often view economic feasibility as attainable only by building large, multi-unit settings. And yet, the larger the size of a congregate project, the greater the risk that it will be perceived as an institution. Chellis et al. states that older persons no longer have the capacity to handle large scale and complex environmental challenges. "To expect them to traverse long corridors (150-200 feet), to manipulate elevators (6-30 floors) and particularly at meals time (previously a family activity), is creating stress, not enhancing the quality of their life" (1982, p. 214).

In sum, congregate housing is a promising model built on the concept of dynamic flexibility and adaptation to the needs of its consumers. It started out, however, responding to the mid-course or central tendencies of the older population rather than on its variability and extreme ranges. Because of the numerical pull of one of these growing extremes in its midst, the very frail, it now runs the risk of being engulfed by the medical and institutional models of services. Congregate housing was created precisely to offer an alternative to those models.

REFERENCES

American Association of Retired Persons (1985). *A Profile of Older Americans.* Washington, DC.

Baldwin, L. (1980). Introduction. In Linda Hubbard (Ed.), *Housing Options for Older Americans.* Washington, DC: American Association of Retired Persons.

Brody, E. (1978). "Community Housing for the Elderly—The Program, the People, the Decision-Making Process and the Research." *Gerontologist,* 18(2) pp. 121-128.

Cantor, M.H. & Donovan, R. (1982). *Enriched Housing: A Viable Alternative for the Frail Elderly.* New York: Fordham University.

Chellis, R.D., Seagle, J. Jr., & Seagle, B.M. (1982). *Congregate Housing for Older People.* Lexington, MA: Lexington Books.

Congregate Housing (1987). Council of State Housing Agencies and National Association of State Units on Aging. Washington, DC.

Cronin, R.C., Drury, M.J., & Gragg, F.E. (1983). *An Evaluation of the FmHA-AoA Demonstration Program of Congregate Housing in Rural Areas Final Report.* Washington, DC: American Institutes for Research.

Department of Health and Human Services (1981). *The 1981 White House Conference on Aging Report on the Mini-Conference on Housing for the Elderly.* Washington, DC.

Donahue, W.T., Thompson, M.M., & Curren, P.J. (1977). *Congregate Housing: An Urgent Need, a Growing Demand.* Washington, DC: International Center for Social Gerontology.

Heumann, L.F. (1976). "Estimating the Local Need for Elderly Congregate Housing." *Gerontologist,* 16(5), 397-403.

Heumann, L. & Brody, D. (1982). *Housing for the Elderly.* New York: St. Martin's.

Kaye, L.W., Monk, A., & Diamond, B.E. (1985). "The Enrichment of Residential Housing Stock for Elderly Tenants: A National Analysis and Case Feasibility Study." Report submitted to the NRTA-AARP Andrus Foundation, Brookdale Institute on Aging and Adult Human Development, Columbia University, New York.

Lawton, M.P. (1980). *Social and Medical Services in Housing for the Aged.* Washington, DC: U.S. Government Printing Office.

_____ (1976). "The Relative Impact of Congregate and Traditional Housing on Elderly Tenants." *Generations,* 16(13).

Longino, C. (1979). "Going Home: Aged Return Migration in the U.S., 1965-1970." *Journal of Gerontology,* 34, 736-745.

Malozemoff, I.K., Anderson, J.G., & Rosenbaum, L.V. (1978). *Housing for the Elderly: Evaluation of the Effectiveness of Congregate Residences.* Boulder, CO: Westview Press.

Monk, A., Kaye, L.W., & Diamond, B.E. (1986). "A Survey Study of Elderly Residents at Brookdale Village." Report Submitted to the Federation of Jewish Philanthropies and the Jewish Association for Services for the Aged. Brookdale Institute on Aging and Adult Human Development, Columbia University, New York.

Nachison, J.S. (1985a). "Who Pays: The Congregate Housing Question." *Generations,* 9(3), 34-37.

_____ (1985b). "Congregate Housing for the Low and Moderate Income Elderly— A Needed Federal State Partnership." *Journal of Housing for the Elderly,* 3(3/4), 65-80.

Newman, S. (1985). "The Shape of Things to Come." *Generations,* 9(3), 14-17.

Pollack, P.B., Higgins, C., Decker, K.C. (1985). *Enriched Housing: A Step-By-Step Program Development Guide.* Unpublished document, Cornell Cooperative Extension Department of Consumer Economics and Housing. New York State Office for the Aging, Rural Aging Services Program Resource Manual 7. Ithaca, NY.

Prosper, V. (1987). "A Review of Congregate Housing in the United States." Report by the New York State Office for the Aging. Albany, NY.

Sherwood, S., Morris, J.N., & Ruchlin, H. (1986). "Alternative Paths to Long-term Care: Nursing Home Geriatric Day Hospital, Senior Center, and Domiciliary Care Options." *American Journal of Public Health,* 76(1) pp. 38-44.

Struyk, R. (1989). "Providing Supportive Services to the Frail Elderly in Federally Assisted Housing." Testimony presented before the Select Committee on Aging, U.S. House of Representatives, May 4 and July 26, 1989. U.S. Government Printing Office, Washington, DC, 1990.

Struyk, R.J. & Soldo, B.J. (1980). *Improving the Elderly's Housing: A Key to Preserving the Nation's Housing Stock and Neighborhood.* Cambridge, MA: Ballinger Publishing Company.

U.S. Congress, House Select Committee on Aging (1988). *Section 202 Housing Budget Crisis.* Washington, DC: U.S. Government Printing Office.

———— (1987). *Dignity, Independence and Cost Effectiveness: The Success of the Congregate Housing Service Programs.* Washington, DC: U.S. Government Printing Office. December.

United States Department of Housing and Urban Development (October 1983). *Monitoring and Technical Assistance Handbook for the Congregate Housing Services Program.* Washington, DC.

I. THEORETICAL PERSPECTIVES

Matching Congregate Housing Settings with a Diverse Elderly Population: Research and Theoretical Considerations

Stephen M. Golant

INTRODUCTION

Many groups are interested in achieving congregate housing accommodations that match or are congruent with the life-styles and needs of older persons. The private sector has obvious motives for trying to develop projects that appeal to a targeted market. Once older people are in their dwellings, managements must regularly decide when to require them to move to more supported living accommodations in their facilities (e.g., to personal care or nursing care units, when available), if and how to provide more supportive services, or when to require their older occupants to leave their projects altogether. The congregate housing residents for their part are concerned that other elderly occupants in their facility (whether new or longtime residents) should have comparable life-styles and activity pat-

Stephen M. Golant, PhD, is Professor in the Department of Geography, University of Florida in Gainsville. His research focuses on the current and future housing situations, service needs, and interregional and intrametropolitan relocation patterns of the U.S. elderly population. He is currently completing a book on the advantages and disadvantages of the housing options currently available to older Americans.

terns. Public housing authorities and nonprofit sponsors of low-rent elderly housing are concerned that their projects, which were originally intended to serve relatively healthy, independent low-income elderly populations, are now being asked to add congregate health facilities to accommodate those older residents who are experiencing a variety of physical and mental impairments. They also must confront the onerous task of deciding when to compel their tenants to leave, because their projects lack appropriate facilities and staff to deal with their elderly population's disabilities. Nonprofit groups involved in the development of shared housing options must not only identify prospective elderly occupants who will benefit from this type of accommodation, but also those who can live together harmoniously. Elderly consumers themselves, not to mention their children, are overwhelmed by the variety of housing options that have suddenly emerged on the market place. They must not only assess which of these options might be best suited to their immediate and long-term needs, but they must also discriminate between honest and unscrupulous sponsors.

Thus a strong rationale exists for understanding the circumstances under which congregate residential settings are likely to be congruent with a diverse population of both existing and prospective elderly occupants. The basic question becomes: when can we expect a good fit or optimum match between older people and their residential environments? This chapter focuses on those research findings and theoretical discussions that have shed light on this question.

THE CONFOUNDING ISSUE OF RELOCATION

The Relocation Experience

Assessing the benefits and the drawbacks of living in congregate housing is complicated because the very act of relocating to this type of facility is itself an experience that impacts on older people's well-being. While this is an issue deserving of its own paper, a few key elements of this problem require identification.

It is well established that older people are more likely to experience unfavorable personal outcomes (e.g., unhappiness, dissatisfaction, anxiety, decline in health) following their residential moves, when they are forced to move involuntarily (e.g., their apartment project is converted to condominiums, or when their poor health makes it impossible for them to live by themselves), when they have not carefully prepared or planned for the move, or when financial constraints or health problems force them to select their new residence from a very limited set of choices (Pastalan, 1983). Thus, even before a new congregate housing residence is initially occupied, older persons may be experiencing anxiety and distress. Indeed, the mere anticipation of moving to alternative quarters may negatively affect an individual's psychological well-being (Tobin & Lieberman, 1976).

Also, a new congregate housing facility is never evaluated on its own terms because it will inevitably be compared with the older person's previous residence. Along with considering how a facility's tangible qualities differ (e.g., smaller size of rooms, better security, better quality of neighborhood, etc.), older persons must also contemplate leaving a home associated with highly significant and irreplaceable personal and family memories and experiences (Golant, 1984a, 1984b; Howell, 1980; O'Bryant, 1983; Rowles, 1983). In stark contrast, an about-to-be occupied congregate housing facility has only a present reality.

Assessments of a congregate housing project will also depend on whether its appearance and features are consistent with an older person's expectations (Campbell, Converse, & Rodgers, 1976). Whatever its virtues, if the reality of a new congregate housing facility falls short of what older people anticipated, then their reactions are more likely to be negative. Thus, whether older people view a new facility as congruent with their needs may in considerable part depend on the accuracy and completeness of earlier received information from family, friends, or marketing agents. This is consistent with other evidence showing that when older people are effectively prepared and counselled about their future accommodations, they cope better with the eventual changes (Yawney & Slover, 1973).

Selection Biases

The reasons that motivate older people to move to a congregate facility in the first place will largely guarantee that its social and physical qualities will match or fit their needs and wants. Much of this "fit" can thereby be explained by a principle found in the "behavior setting" theory of Barker (1968). Simply stated: people purposively select environments and environments purposively select people.

What this means is that elderly people will decide on a place to move because it has qualities (e.g., health or social services, leisure and recreational opportunities, design features, and staff attitudes) that are consistent with their present or expected life-styles, health status and financial resources. For their part, congregate housing managements impose criteria (however informal or formalized these might be) by which they decide whether older people can *enter* or *remain* in their facilities (Hiatt, 1982). Besides financial status, these considerations usually are based on the older person's physical and mental health, involving observations and assessments of mental clarity and alertness, eccentric behaviors, sensory impairments (seeing, hearing abilities), capacity for self-care, mobility, and diet needs. These assessments may be conducted either by the in-house staff of the congregate housing facility or by outside professionals (e.g., private physicians). In the case of elderly persons already living in a facility, it may be the other elderly occupants who call attention to deviations in these "understood" criteria. The management further controls who remains and who stays by its willingness to provide new services or benefits to accommodate those older residents with emerging disabilities. The older residents themselves may play a crucial role by serving as "helpers" or resource persons to the more vulnerable elderly tenants, thereby delaying their departure to more supportive facilities.

Allowing only those occupants with certain personal habits may also impose subtle influences on the atmosphere of the congregate housing complex. In my own community, an adult congregate living facility does not allow alcohol to be consumed in any of its public areas, including the dining room. While genuinely inspired by religious beliefs, this rule will obviously "turn off" a certain group of prospective elderly occupants, even as it attracts others.

While these selection biases increase the likelihood of a fit between elderly residents and their congregate settings (Kasl & Rosenfield, 1980), "mismatches" will inevitably result for the following reasons:

1. When older people's prior information about the congregate housing option has been incomplete or inaccurate and the facility turns out to be different than what was originally presented.
2. When individual preferences are not completely realized by the qualities of the congregate housing facility, but personal constraints such as a limited income, or a need to live close to family members, still make it the "best choice."
3. When older occupants living in a facility experience unexpected changes in their personal resources (e.g., health, income) or lifestyles (e.g., new leisure pursuits, the death of a spouse) that cannot be accommodated by the residential setting.
4. When the environment of the residential setting changes in some divergent and unexpected fashion (e.g., such as might occur when a congregate facility experiences a change in ownership or management or incurs financial difficulties).

Even as we recognize the importance of knowing the circumstances underlying the moving decisions of older people, we unfortunately have less than perfect understanding of the relocation deliberations of at least three distinctive groups of older people: (a) elderly persons who were interested in the idea of congregate living but who subsequently opted not to move to this housing option, because it was considered inappropriate for their life-styles or needs, it was unavailable when needed, or because disability or death prevented a planned occupancy; (b) elderly persons who earlier left a facility because either they or the management believed it did not suit their needs; (c) elderly persons who were living in a facility that was unresponsive to their needs, but who have since died.

Identifying and studying these three elderly groups will obviously be difficult. Yet an understanding of their decision-making may provide some of the best insights into why older people sometimes consider congregate housing to be an inappropriate place to live.

OLDER PEOPLE BECOME THE ENVIRONMENT

Even as mismatches sometimes occur, the above individual- and environmental-selecting mechanisms usually result in a particular congregate housing facility being occupied by older persons who are more alike than they are different. The uniformity of their attitudes, values, and behaviors will in turn influence the day-to-day operation of the residential setting. Having "inappropriate" staff fired, modifying the rules of the management, and creating pressure on the administration to modify features of the setting are some of the practical outcomes. Moreover, an aggregation of relatively homogeneous older persons will influence the overall image of the congregate housing setting. Thus, when the elderly residents are active and independent, the residential setting becomes defined as "active" and "independent." Conversely, a residential setting occupied by a very old, more vulnerable, and sedentary elderly population becomes identified in these terms.

The owners and management of adult congregate living facilities are not insensitive to the practical implications of the Barker principle. Often wanting their facility to be known as the home of the vigorous "young-old," they are wary about providing elderly residents who live in independent living quarters with too many supportive services. They fear that such a response will foster a "dependent" image of their settings resulting in selective shunning of their sites by prospective elderly tenants who are active and independent (Merrill & Hunt, 1990). Importantly, the issue then shifts from that of whether there is a people-environment match in the congregate housing facility, to *whether the "match" itself is desirable and consistent with the organizational goals of the owner or management*.

This very issue is now being confronted by the operators of this country's low-income public housing projects (Holshouser, 1988). Whereas these projects were originally occupied by nonelderly tenants in the instance of family housing or by the "young-old" elderly in the instance of senior-citizen housing, many of these facilities have now become the homes of the "old-old" (i.e., over the age of 75). Opting not to move, their residents have literally aged-in-place. The result is an increased need by these tenants of medical and social services that were not originally envisioned for these housing projects. While the management often recognizes that their elderly occupants require a more supportive living situation, at issue is to what extent the "low-rent housing facility" should be transformed in order to achieve this people-environment match or congruence. Alternatively, should "congruence" be achieved by requiring that these more "dependent" elderly move elsewhere?

THE DEPICTION OF THE CONGREGATE FACILITY'S ENVIRONMENT

The Complexity of the Task

Assessments of whether a congregate housing facility does provide an appropriate environment for its elderly occupants will only be as effective as portrayals of its attributes and qualities are relevant, complete and accurate. The residential environment of older people is now usually characterized in very broad terms (e.g., Golant, 1984b; Lawton, 1980; Moos & Lemke, 1985). It encompasses not only the dwelling units and buildings (including their grounds) of the project, but also the neighborhood, community, and even the state and region in which these are located. Researchers have described these settings with respect to their natural features (e.g., temperature, precipitation, insect problems), architectural components (e.g., building type, design, appliances, floor layout, color selections), transportation accessibility, urban qualities (e.g., traffic congestion, crime), service availability, interpersonal relationships (e.g., availability of friends, family), social situation (e.g., overall population composition of building or neighborhood as indicated by its mix of age, sex, ethnic, racial, marital status, and economic characteristics), legal and administrative aspects (e.g., state regulations pertaining to congregate housing, Supplemental Security Income eligibility, amount and availability of Medicaid funding), and program and organizational features (e.g., rules and regulations of a congregate housing facility).

The seemingly infinite ways to describe a residential setting has resulted in environmental classifications that lack consistency and uniformity. The complexity of this cataloguing task is illustrated by the possible depictions of the deceptively straightforward quality, "amount of privacy." There is "visual" privacy (a private place where an older person escapes from the public view), "auditory" privacy (a private place where an older person can talk or converse without being heard), "interpersonal" privacy (a place where an older person can watch and listen but not involve herself or himself in the conversation or activity), and "administrative" privacy, whereby some or all aspects of an older person's life are protected from scrutiny from a congregate housing management.

The environment is depicted not only in terms of what it contains but also whether these contents are in some sense "good" or "bad." On the positive side, the residential environment is conceptualized in terms of its resources, its incentives, its supportive, stimulating and motivating aspects, or its potential for fulfilling older people's needs. On the negative side, it is conceptualized in terms of its constraints, its limitations, its disincentives, or its potential for preventing older people from realizing their needs.

Because of a congregate housing project's diverse content and varied potentials, its position along multiple continuums of opposing (i.e., good-bad) environmental dimensions must be established. Representative descriptive and evaluative scales include: expensive-inexpensive (with respect to entry and/or monthly fees), for profit-nonprofit sponsorship, structured-unstructured (i.e., its institutional vs. noninstitutional organizational qualities), independent-dependent (with respect to its residents' composition), tolerant-intolerant (with respect to management's response to diverse or deviant behaviors), sparseness-richness (with respect to its staff and services), constant-accommodating (with respect to the changeability of its programs, services, design features), sociable-unsociable (with respect to the residents' friendliness), responsive-unresponsive (with respect to management's reaction to tenant needs), stimulating-unstimulating (with respect to its offered activities and programs), and design sensitive-design insensitive (with respect to its architectural features) (Pincus, 1968; Lemke & Moos, 1989; Golant, 1980, 1984b; Kahana, 1974; Lawton, 1977; Nehrke et al., 1984). Thus, at any one time, a congregate housing facility may contain features that both facilitate and block human needs or benefit and harm its occupants. For example, even as a low-rent senior citizens' congregate housing project relieves its occupants of financial concerns and meal preparation, its age-segregated status may impose an incompatible social situation on those elderly tenants who have usually culled their friendships from the young and who dislike living with older people (Golant, 1980; Rosow, 1967).

If in fact an environment may be congruent in some respects, but incongruent in others (Kahana, Liang, & Felton, 1980; Moos & Lemke, 1985), then the issue becomes whether different aspects of the residential setting should be assigned equal weight or salience when considering their impact. For example, an aspect of where one lives (living far from a family member) may be disagreeable (incongruent with person's needs), but it may not be deemed very significant in one's everyday affairs. Most research efforts have skirted this issue. An exception is the research of Nehrke et al. (1984) on Veterans Administration's domiciliary facilities, which weighted the older occupants' environmental assessments on the basis of their expressions of "felt importance."

The task of describing the congregate housing setting is further complicated because it often encompasses several distinctive spatial zones, each of which may be assigned very different positions along any environmental quality continuum (Golant, 1984b). This is exemplified by the classic study of Carp (1966), whereby she assessed the impact of a new public housing environment on its older occupants. While their apartment units were positively evaluated, the elderly tenants had reservations about their neighborhood because it was located in a distressed area of the city and was inconvenient to shopping facilities. Another example is provided by inner city apartment hotels containing single room occupancy units (SROs). While the apartment units themselves are described as internally secure from intruders, their neighborhoods often suffer from very high crime rates (Franck, 1989). Textbook attempts to categorize the continuing care retirement community along an independent-institutional continuum are misleading for a similar reason. Such a facility often contains a set of very distinctive living areas ranging from ordinary independent apartment units to personal care units and nursing care centers. And whereas the independent apartments may be considered well-run, the nursing care center may be managed poorly. Even the apparently unambiguous designation of a congregate housing facility's "personal care or assisted care" wing may be misleading. Some administrators allow physically and mentally impaired elderly persons requiring skilled nursing care to remain in their personal care units if the occupants can afford a full-time private registered nurse.

Beyond the issue of diversity, neatly aligning an attribute of a residential setting along a "good-bad" continuum has proved to be more difficult than expected in real world applications. The research of Kahana, Liang, and Felton (1980), extending the work of French, Rodgers, and Cobb (1974), for example, emphasized that whether some quality of the residential setting is construed as being positive or negative will depend on the extent of its presence. In laypersons' terms, the expressions "too much of a good thing" or "not enough of a good thing" captures the essence of this idea. This implies that to speak of a residential setting as supportive, quiet and offering privacy may say very little about its desirability, if it offers too much help, too much quiet, or too much privacy.

This dilemma is illustrated by attempts to distinguish a residential setting as "good" or "bad" on the basis of whether it provides a physically, socially, and psychologically "secure" environment. It is agreed that achieving a secure place to live is one motive for older persons seeking congregate housing facilities. However, even as an administrator establishes a more secure housing setting—perhaps by having staff members more carefully monitor the residents—there is a risk of creating such an overly protected environment that some elderly residents feel that the management is violating their privacy or independence.

It quickly becomes apparent that what constitutes a desirable or attractive congregate housing feature depends very much on who is doing the judging. With the exception of housing projects that are in extreme states of disrepair, grossly mismanaged, or blatantly insensitive to the concerns of their elderly occupants, there are few absolutes with respect to the appropriateness of a congregate housing facility's qualities. Some families find this housing option to be highly attractive; others are repulsed by this type of accommodations. "Experts" tend to identify more design flaws in congregate housing facilities than the older occupants themselves (Brennan, Moos, & Lemke, 1988). Elderly residents and management also find reason to disagree. For example, while the older resident who suddenly becomes physically impaired would benefit from services delivered inside her apartment, the management might view such a policy as inconsistent with the "independent living" image of the congregate housing project.

Researchers themselves cannot agree as to who should judge a residential setting's quality of life. Some studies depend on evaluations of the staff or administrators (e.g., Kahana, Liang, & Felton, 1980); others depend on the environmental assessments of the elderly residents (Nehrke et al., 1984); while still others use a combination of resident reports, staff assessments, and outside observers (Lemke and Moos, 1985). Nor should the role of researchers be underestimated. By their categorizations and measurements of an environment's features or qualities, they can significantly influence conclusions about an environment's impact. In short, researchers are not value-free. Their views are often biased by their academic specialties or their own idiosyncratic views (Golant, 1984b).

CONGRUENCE AND THE DIVERSITY
OF THE ELDERLY POPULATION

Varied Approaches

Both theoretical treatments and actual research findings have argued that older persons living in the very same congregate housing project will react differently to its attributes. What is considered by one older person to be an attractive feature will be considered by another as a nuisance; what is viewed as organizational efficiency by some will be considered overly bureaucratic by others; what will stimulate one older person will stress out another. Consequently, where a residential feature is positioned along a good-to-bad or supportive-to-unsupportive continuum will depend much on the characteristics of the elderly persons relating to them. How old people judge the quality of their congregate housing settings is inseparably linked to their perceptions, thoughts, and actions (Golant, 1984b).

While consensus exists that the very same qualities of a residential setting will impinge differently on the well-being of its older occupants, what constitutes an individual's "well-being" has varied from study to study (Kasl & Rosenfield, 1980). The most frequently defined measures have included: (a) intrapsychic or inner individual states such as mood, self-concept, morale, life satisfaction, apathy, depression, hostility, alienation; (b) physical or psychophysiological individual symptoms such as fatigue, headaches, poor appetite, poor health, days in bed; (c) individual performance measures such as the ability to carry out the everyday tasks of daily living and home management activities without assistance or the number of days of restricted activity; (d) social activity patterns such as the extent and significance of friendship, neighbor and family contacts and organizational or group memberships of the elderly person; and (e) evaluations or feelings expressed by the older person about particular residential qualities, as indicated by expressions of satisfaction, pride, fear, need for service, and loneliness.

Researchers have also varied notably as to how they have conceptualized and measured the individual basis for older people's differing responses to where they live. At the risk of oversimplifying, researchers focusing on this question can be divided into two groups. There are those who have treated the elderly person as a highly complex human being or "whole person" with multiple dispositions, traits, behaviors, and complex backgrounds (Kahana, 1974; Carp & Carp, 1984; Rowles, 1983; Golant, 1984b); and there are those who, while recognizing this complexity, have emphasized one or more characteristics of the person considered central to all their environmental transactions (e.g., Lawton, 1989; Parmelee & Lawton, 1990; Regnier, 1981). We focus first on the latter approach.

Competence as the Basis for Individual Diversity

A preponderance of attention has been focused on the varying competence levels of older people, that is, on the extent to which they are able to perform acceptably (according to agreed-upon societal standards) a full range of everyday covert (e.g., thinking, perceiving, negotiating, problem-solving) and overt (e.g., taking care of oneself, taking care of one's home, going outside, taking a walk, manipulating an oven's controls) behaviors.

Defining and measuring "incompetence" is itself a thorny problem for the administrators of the congregate housing facility. Procedures by which independent functioning is assessed and the extent to which these are formalized (i.e., recorded as part of published rules and regulations) vary considerably among facilities. While very serious impairments are simple enough to document, in many instances older people border between being able to remain in their independent units and needing a more supportive personal care setting. Complicating the issue are attempts by older people to disguise their disabilities, sometimes aided in their efforts by the assistance of other concerned residents.

Assessments of competence are often restricted to the activities and performance of the elderly *individual*. Yet in many instances, older persons themselves do not conceive of their capabilities in this narrow fashion. Rather, competence is viewed in conjunction with the resources of another person. Many married older persons, for example, are confident that they can rely on their spouses to assist them (if and when necessary) with their usual activities of daily living and home management tasks. They take comfort in knowing that there is someone available for them to share both their emotional highs and lows. Other older persons have confidence that such instrumental and emotional supports will be forthcoming from other family members or even from an extremely close friend or neighbor. Because they firmly and confidently hold these beliefs (whatever their actual validity), the conception of their own competence becomes inseparably linked with the personal resources of these "significant others." The existence of such interindividual alliances helps to explain why the death or institutionalization of a "significant other" may constitute such a devastating experience for an older person. It is often as if part of the individual's basis for autonomy has been ripped away. Congregate housing administrators often are confronted with the dilemma of how to respond to a husband-wife older couple, one of whom has become too dependent to remain in the facility's independent units. Their actions inevitably depend on whether more supportive accommodations or personal care services are available in the facility, if the couple can financially afford these "separate" accommodations (i.e., one spouse in the independent unit, the other in the personal care facility), and if private in-home assistance is feasible and affordable.

Competence and Environmental Congruence

In two related propositions, Lawton (1989) has theorized about how the impact of a residential environment will depend on the older person's level of competence. First, "the environmental docility hypothesis" argued that as the competence of older persons declines, a greater proportion of their behavioral outcomes will be explained by the attributes of their environments. Expressed somewhat differently, older persons with lower or declining levels of competence will be more susceptible to the vagaries of their residential settings than those with higher or stable competence levels. For instance, because I am frail, I am less willing to risk falling on a slippery sidewalk after it rains and I will remain in my house until the sidewalk dries. The implication: equally noxious residential qualities will not lead to all elderly persons experiencing the same likelihood or extent of negative outcomes.

Second, the "environmental proactivity hypothesis" argued that "as the person becomes more competent, the environment affords increasing resources relevant to the person's needs" (Lawton, 1989, p. 140). In other words, as the competence of older people improves, so also does their awareness of the resources and potentialities of their surroundings and their ability to shape, manipulate, or utilize these to their own advantage and satisfaction (see also Golant, 1984a, pp. 263-265).

The apparent straightforwardness of the above propositions, however, masks the complexities of achieving residential settings that are consistent with their elderly occupants' capacities. For example, it is possible for a congregate housing staff to be overly responsive to the needs of their elderly residents. Lawton (1985, p. 459) has argued that the "environmental demands on the more competent may become reduced to the point where their skills are not sufficiently exercised.'' He points to the service-rich congregate housing setting that may encourage ''passive contentment,'' implying an individual's decreased involvement with the people and activities outside his or her congregate housing complex. Langer's (1983, p. 285) arguments are relevant here even though they were raised in connection with older people in nursing homes:

> . . . Simply helping people may make them incompetent. While meaning well, it communicates to the person that he or she is not able to do whatever it is for him- or herself. If the person faces no difficulty, if there are no challenges, large or small, feelings of mastery are precluded and consequences such as involution, depression, and premature death are real possibilities rather than mere exaggeration. Helping the resident to get dressed to go to breakfast (either out of concern for the resident or to save time for the staff) may only result in feelings of incompetence and dependence for the resident and ultimately take more of the staff's time, since the individual will soon come to assume the need for such help.

On the other hand, an emphasis on autonomous or independent living in a congregate housing setting may not be in the best interests of its more vulnerable elderly occupants. Lemke and Moos (1989, S146) have argued that whereas more competent or ''high functioning residents are more active in settings where other residents are active, functionally able, and have more social resources and where autonomy is greater,'' the ''very impaired residents in such settings may experience negative effects of a too-demanding environment, with reductions in their self-initiated activity to below the level found for similarly impaired residents in less demanding environments.'' They propose that such incongruent resident situations be alleviated by increasing the amount of staff counseling and involvement with the less competent elderly residents.

Private developers are also sometimes frustrated in their attempts to fill their congregate housing projects with older people they consider to have appropriate competence levels. Even as they do their best to market their projects to ''young-old'' elderly persons, this group often avoids these facilities because they are seen as offering too supportive of an environment. One example: the congregate dining room facility in which two or even three meals a day are provided as part of the monthly ''rent.'' Paradoxically, even as this service is positively portrayed as an amenity that typifies resort living, some prospective elderly residents think otherwise. Being able to prepare their own meals is for them the single most important behavior from which they derive confidence in their ability to live independently. Thus the "necessity" of partaking of congregate meals will be construed as a negative feature.

One solution to the dilemma of trying to appeal to an older population with diverse capacities is to make the congregate housing environment as flexible as possible. This implies giving elderly residents an array of features and services from which to choose. In response, an increasing number of congregate housing facilities and continuing care retirement communities have "unbundled" their service packages. By this practice older occupants are given the flexibility of selecting and paying only for those services and features that they currently consider most central to their needs.

Even with such choices, Parmelee and Lawton (1990, p. 468) suggest that attempts by congregate housing residents to achieve simultaneously both security and autonomy may be an elusive goal.

> Gains in security, in the form of increased access to health care and other services, a more manageable environment, and a relatively dense social-supportive environment, are achieved at the cost of some loss of choice and independence.

In short, older occupants in these housing settings will only benefit from some of its features by giving up their rights to others.

A "Whole Person" Perspective

While a focus on an older occupant's competence is important, it is but one of a myriad of individual differences influencing the "fittingness" of the congregate housing environment. Gerontologists have identified a wide array of other personal attributes that are likely to underlie an environment's impact (Golant, 1984b). The congregate housing experience has variously been linked to: a person's need and willingness to associate with persons of similar social identity (i.e., to live with other persons of similar ethnic, religious, racial, or class backgrounds); patterns of age identification (i.e., whether older people hold positive attitudes towards living with other older people); individual needs for privacy, control, order (or regularity), and novelty; an individual's current psychological well-being (i.e., an older person who is overall more happy with her life will evaluate her surroundings more positively); an individual's adaptation level (i.e., a life-time of salient past housing experiences will be brought to bear on present residential assessments); and individual expectation levels (i.e., what kinds of standards are held by the individual).

An unresolved issue is how to weight the relative importance of these individual differences. For example, do judgments of the appropriateness of a congregate housing option more strongly reflect an individual's personality make-up (e.g., a need to dominate others) or an inability to live independently? How are conflicting individual dispositions to be interpreted (e.g., repulsion of living in age-segregated living arrangements but a need to feel secure)? There is also disagreement as to whether differences in the way older people react to the congregate housing environment reflect life-long patterns as opposed to recent events accompanying old age (McCrae & Costa, 1984). For example, how is the congregate housing environment viewed differently by the elderly woman who was widowed at the age of 30 as opposed to the elderly woman who lost her husband only a year ago; and by the older person who was disabled in young adulthood as opposed to the older person who became impaired only after retirement?

WHAT TO MANIPULATE?

This paper has emphasized that the attributes of both the individual and the residential environment together account for whether a congregate housing setting will be a "good match" with current or prospective elderly residents. Thus, to change the environmental outcomes experienced by older people, interventions can occur at either the individual or environmental level. Through individual or group counselling we can try to modify or change older people's attitudes and behaviors so that they can appreciate the potential of congregate living or that they can deal more effectively with where they currently live. Alternatively, we can change or modify the residential settings of older people so as to alleviate or eliminate those environmental aspects that appear to be the greatest sources of dissatisfaction or discomfort.

Whatever our strategy, we must recognize that our ability to change outcomes will be constrained. There will be limits beyond which additional environmental modifications will have minimal impact on elderly behaviors and more individual counselling will not make older people more comfortable and adept in their surroundings. Residential settings designed, organized and administered to achieve specific goals can only be manipulated successfully up to a certain point. It is then the task of the professional, the planner, and the administrator to recognize their potentialities for effecting these positive outcomes through their awareness and understanding of how older people relate to their surroundings and how the surroundings impinge on their older occupants.

We clearly have the know-how to improve the quality of older people's lives and residential settings. We should not be surprised, however, if our increments do not constitute giant but tiny steps. We often do not appreciate the positive impact of a multitude of small changes.

REFERENCES

Barker, R. (1968). *Ecological Psychology*. Stanford, CA: Stanford University Press.

Brennan, P. L., Moos, R. L., & Lemke, S. (1988). Preferences of older adults and experts for physical and architectural features of group living facilities. *The Gerontologist*, 28, pp. 84-90.

Campbell, A., Converse, P. G., & Rodgers, W. (1976). *The Quality of American Life*. NY: Russell Sage.

Carp, F. M. (1966). *A Future for the Aged*. Austin: University of Texas Press.

Carp, F. M. & Carp, A. (1984). A complementary/congruence model of well-being or mental health for the community elderly. In I. Altman, M. P. Lawton, & J. Wohlwill (Eds.), *Elderly People and the Environment*. NY: Plenum, pp. 279-336.

Franck, K. A. (1989). Single room occupancy housing. In K. A. Franck & S. Ahrentzen (Eds.), *New Households, New Housing*. NY: Van Nostrand Reinhold, pp. 245-262.

French, J. R., Rodgers, W., & Cobb, S. (1974). Adjustment as person-environment fit. In G. V. Coelho, D. A. Hamburg, & J. E. Adams (Eds.), *Coping and Adaptation*. NY: Basic Books, pp. 316-333.

Golant, S. M. (1980). Locational-environmental perspectives on old-age segregated residential areas in the United States. In D. T. Herbert & R. J. Johnston (Eds.), *Geography and the Urban Environment*. Vol. 3. London: Wiley, pp. 257-294.

Golant, S. M. (1984a). The effects of residential and activity behaviors on old people's environmental experiences. In I. Altman, M. P. Lawton, & J. Wohlwill (Eds.), *Elderly People and the Environment*. NY: Plenum, pp. 239-278.

Golant, S. M. (1984b). *A Place to Grow Old*. NY: Columbia University Press.

Helson, H. (1964). *Adaptation-Level Theory*. NY: Harper & Row.

Hiatt, L. G. 1982. Grouping elders of different abilities. In R. D. Chellis, J. F. Seagle & B. M. Seagle (Eds.), *Congregate Housing for Older People*. Lexington, MA: D. C. Heath & Co., pp. 27-49.

Holshouser, Jr., W. L. (1988). *Aging in Place: The Demographics and Service Needs of Elders in Urban Public Housing*. Boston: Citizens Housing and Planning Association, 1988.

Howell, S. C. (1980). Environments as hypotheses in human aging research. In L. Poon (Ed.), *Aging in the 1980s: Psychological Issues*. Washington, DC: American Psychological Association, pp. 424-432.

Kahana, E. (1974). Matching environment to needs of the aged: A conceptual scheme. In J. F. Gubrium (Ed.), *Late Life: Recent Developments in the Sociology of Aging*. Springfield, IL: Thomas, 1974.

Kahana, E., Liang, J., & Felton (1980). Alternative models of person-environment fit: Prediction of morale in three homes for the aged. *Journal of Gerontology*, 35, pp. 584-595.

Kasl, S. V. & Rosenfield, S. (1980). The residential environment and its impact on the mental health of the aged. In J. E. Birren & R. B. Sloane (Eds.), *Handbook of Mental Health and Aging*. NY: Prentice-Hall, pp. 468-498.

Langer, E. J. (1983). *The Psychology of Control*. Beverly Hills, CA: Sage.

Lawton, M. P. (1977). The impact of the environment on aging and behavior. In J. E. Birren & K. W. Schaie (Eds.), *Handbook of the Psychology of Aging*. NY: Van Nostrand Reinhold, 1977, pp. 276-301.

Lawton, M. P. (1980). *Environment and Aging*. Monterey, CA: Brooks/Cole.

Lawton, M. P. (1985). Housing and living environments of older people. In R. H. Binstock & E. Shanas (Eds.), *Handbook of Aging and the Social Sciences* (Second Edition). NY: Van Nostrand Reinhold, pp. 450-478.

Lawton, M. P. (1989). Environmental proactivity and affect in older people. In S. Spacapan & S. Oskamp (Eds.), *The Social Psychology of Aging*. Newbury Park, CA: Sage, 1989, pp. 135-163.

Lemke, S. & Moos, R. H. (1989). Personal and environmental determinants of activity involvement among elderly residents of congregate facilities. *Journal of Gerontology: Social Sciences*, 44, pp. S139-S148.

McCrae, R. R. & Costa, P. T. (1984). *Emerging Lives, Enduring Dispositions*. Boston: Little, Brown.

Merrill, J., & Hunt, M. E. (1990). Aging in place: A dilemma for retirement housing administrators. *Journal of Applied Gerontology*, 9, pp. 60-76.

Moos, R. H., & Lemke, S. (1985). Specialized living environments for older people. In J. Birren & K. W. Schaie (Eds.), *Handbook of the Psychology of Aging* (Second Edition). NY: Van Nostrand Reinhold, pp. 864-887.

Nehrke, M. F. et al., (1984). Differences in person-environment congruence between microenvironments. *Canadian Journal of Aging*, 3, pp. 117-132.

O'Bryant, S. L. (1983). The subjective value of "home" to older homeowners. *Journal of Housing for the Elderly*, 1, 29-43.

Parmelee, P. A. & Lawton, M. P. (1990). The design of special environments for the aged. In J. Birren & K. W. Schaie (Eds.), *Handbook of the Psychology of Aging* (Third Edition). San Diego: Academic Press, pp. 464-488.

Pastalen, L. A. (1983). Environmental displacement. In G. D. Rowles & R. J. Ohta (Eds.), *Aging and Milieu*. New York: Academic Press, pp. 189-203.

Pincus, A. (1968). The definition and measurement of the institutional environment in homes for the aged. *The Gerontologist*, 8, pp. 207-210.

Regnier, V. (1981). Neighborhood images and use: A case study. In M. P. Lawton & S. Hoover (Eds.), *Community Housing Choices for Older Americans*. NY: Springer, pp. 180-197.

Rosow, I. (1967). *Social Integration of the Aged*. NY: Free Press.

Rowles, G. D. (1983). Place and personal identity in old age: Observations from Appalachia. *Journal of Environmental Psychology*, 3, pp. 219-313.

Scheidt, R. J. & Windley, P. G. (1985). The ecology of aging. In J. Birren & K. W. Schaie (Eds.), *Handbook of Psychology of Aging* (Second Edition). NY: Van Nostrand Reinhold, pp. 245-258.

Tobin, S. S. & Lieberman, M. A. (1976). *Last Home for the Aged*. San Francisco: Jossey-Bass.

Yawney, B. A. & Slover, D. L. (1973). Relocation of the elderly. *Social Work*, 3, pp. 86-95.

II. POLICY PERSPECTIVES

Housing Policy in the United States: Trends, Future Needs, and Implications for Congregate Housing

G. Thomas Kingsley
Raymond J. Struyk

The early 1990s are likely to be an extremely important time in the continuing evolution of U.S. housing policy. Indeed, many cognoscenti expect that major reform legislation will be enacted by the Congress in 1990 or 1991. Why is there such pressure for change and what might the changes mean for housing for the elderly?

G. Thomas Kingsley, MCP, is Director of the Urban Institute's Center for Public Finance and Housing. He is a senior planner and program manager whose career has focused on the analysis, planning, financing and management of urban development both internationally and within the United States. His major publications include Urban Economics and National Development (with George E. Peterson), and the Cleveland Metropolitan Economy (with A. S. Gurwitz). Raymond J. Struyk, PhD, is Director of The Urban Institute's International Activities Center. An economist, he is a widely recognized expert on housing and urban development problems in developing nations and in the United States. His major publications include Housing for the Elderly in 2010: Projections and Policy Options (with S. Newman and H. Katsura), and Future U. S. Housing Policy: Meeting the Demographic Challenge (with M. A. Turner and M. Ueno).

This paper briefly addresses these large questions. To do so, however, requires that we examine the forces demanding change, and take careful stock of some important trends in policy development and of current housing policy and associated government actions.

The United States, through legislation, has established an extremely ambitious set of policy goals, which have been summarized by Downs (1988) as follows:

- "Realization as soon as feasible of . . . a decent home and a suitable living environment for every American Family";
- Providing housing assistance to low-income households as well as to certain specific groups—the elderly, Indians, disabled veterans, persons displaced by government action—so that they can occupy decent and affordable housing;
- Encouraging homeownership among households, regardless of their incomes;
- Increasing the total available supply of decent-quality housing units of all types and at all price levels;
- Eliminating racial and ethnic discrimination in housing markets;
- Stimulating the economy by increasing construction activity in the housing industry;
- Improving the quality of deteriorated neighborhoods; and
- Reducing the concentration of low-income households in poverty areas.

Importantly for the elderly, an additional goal is gradually becoming part of this more traditional list: Enabling the frail elderly, the physically impaired, and the chronically mentally ill to remain in the community as long as feasible.

A veritable arsenal of programs (summarized later) has been created to help attain these goals. These numerous programs neither were created in a single period of legislative activity nor have they been steadily added over the years. Rather they have been created in several bursts spread over the last half century.

By 1980, it appeared that priority given to housing goals was diminishing. But as the decade unfolded, several new trends once again raised concern about housing issues in national policy debates. Four developments over recent years particularly stand out:

- The second half of the 1980s witnessed a "threat to the American dream," with a two percentage point decline in the overall rate of homeownership and greater declines for younger households;
- The combination of rent levels rising faster than general inflation coupled with a growing number of poor households caused the majority of poor households to spend over 30 percent of their cash incomes on housing and a significant minority to spend more than half;
- Homelessness by an estimated half million Americans every night became a highly visible symbol of the gap between the lofty goals of housing policy and its reality for some Americans; and,
- The persistence of poverty among inner-city residents and the belief that more creative and effective public intervention must be devised, including the use of housing assistance as an incentive for encouraging persons to join the economic mainstream.

In part to address these causes and in part to deal with more fundamental problems, the Congress is likely to write major legislation. Senators Cranston and D'Amato began an elaborate process to develop reform legislation in 1987 and introduced an omnibus bill in 1989. Congressman Gonzalez, Chair of the housing subcommittee of the House Committee on Banking, Housing and Urban Affairs introduced a very different omnibus bill in early 1990. And the Administration has submitted its package of ambitious new legislative initiatives developed by HUD Secretary Jack Kemp.

In this paper we first briefly summarize the major episodes in U.S. housing policy, with particular emphasis on the 1980s. We then hazard a look at the future — initially for housing policy in general and then for policies affecting the independent elderly, especially the frail elderly.

INITIATING THE FEDERAL ROLE

The federal government had virtually no direct involvement in housing until the 1930s, when conditions of the great depression heightened nation-wide concern for housing issues. During that decade it initiated the three approaches that still remain as the basic vehicles of national housing policy:

1. Facilitating the workings of the housing finance system.
2. Providing housing assistance to lower-income households through public housing and other means.
3. Creating housing-oriented incentives in the federal tax code.

Figure 1 summarizes changes in the way these approaches have been applied since then and the major factors that motivated those shifts. Clearly, the spotlight has moved from one approach to another over the decades.

In the 1930s, the first approach was dominant. As a response to the devastation of housing finance during the depression, the nation established: (1) the Federal Housing Administration (FHA), which provided insurance for long-term low down payment mortgages, significantly reducing the risk of loans for housing; (2) the Federal National Mortgage Association (FNMA), which further reduced that risk by providing a secondary mortgage market; and (3) the Federal Home Loan Bank (FHLB), which regulated the lenders and provided them with a central source of credit.

While this system was put in place in the 1930s, its benefits were not quantitatively significant until it addressed the post World War II housing shortage. This era is generally regarded as the period of America's greatest success in housing.[1] The system promoted mortgage lending that was much more stable and much less expensive than had existed before 1930, and thus laid the base for the boom in single-family home construction that stretched from the late 1940s through the 1950s.

As impressive as they were, however, these changes did not directly address the housing conditions of the poor. The deplorable state of low income housing in the depression years and before motivated the federal government's first venture into the second of its three approaches: the public housing program, created by the Housing Act of 1937. Through this program, public housing is built and operated by local public housing authorities but federal subsidies cover the full cost of project development. (In the initial program design, operating costs were to be covered by tenant rent payments, although federal support on that side was also required later in the program's evolution.) Annual net additions to the stock of public housing averaged 27,700 units over the 1950s and 41,500 over the 1960s — impressive growth, but the totals remained quite small in relation to total net additions to the U.S. occupied housing stock (an average of 1.03 million units per year over those two decades).[2]

Figure 1
EVOLUTION OF FEDERAL HOUSING POLICY

	1930s	late 1940s to 1950s	1960s to mid 1970s	Late 1970s to 1980s
Circumstances	Great Depression •high unemployment •bank failures and foreclosures •lack of long-term mortgage financing	Postwar housing shortage •rapid household formation •rapid income growth	Persistence of poverty •central city decline •shortage of low-cost housing	Reassessment •high inflation •near collapse of thrift institutions •high costs of subsidized housing •improved housing conditions •proliferation of tax shelters
Policy responses	Highly regulated system of housing finance to mobilize mortgage funds, boost housing production, generate employment	High volume of mortgage insurance to enable newly forming households to buy single-family, suburban homes Tax benefits for home ownership	Rent subsidies, financing and tax benefits to generate production of low-cost rental housing	Deregulation of housing finances Tax reform Shift from subsidized housing production to vouchers

From the 1950s to the present, the most important embodiment of the third approach has been allowing homeowners to deduct mortgage interest payments from their income for tax purposes (more will be said about this later).

CHANGING EMPHASES IN THE 1960s AND 1970s

The 1960s and 1970s saw considerable further growth of federal involvement in housing policy, particularly in assistance to low income groups. A new type of program directed toward that end was started in 1961 — publicly assisted housing. Publicly assisted housing projects are built and operated by private developers but federal subsidies enable the owner to provide units to low- and moderate-income households at reduced rents. The theory was that publicly assisted housing would add to the total output of low rent housing, and serve those whose incomes were inadequate to allow them to pay market rents but higher than the target group for public housing.[3]

The nation's support for federal housing assistance probably reached its high point later in the decade when the Kaiser Committee (President's Committee on Urban Housing, 1969) called for a stronger national commitment to improving the housing conditions of the poor. The creation of the U.S. Department of Housing and Urban Development (HUD) in 1968 was also an important symbol in this regard. And the public and publicly assisted housing programs responded with record construction volumes in the early 1970s.

But these programs were evidencing problems even then — problems President Nixon judged serious enough to cause him to place a moratorium on further production in 1973. In the Housing and Community Development Act of 1974, Congress created a new form of publicly assisted housing in part designed to try to correct the ills of earlier versions. But by the end of the decade, federal production programs had lost much of their support. The most prominent explanations were:

1. The production programs had proved extremely expensive. The *annual* subsidy cost of publicly assisted housing (including interest rate subsidies and tax benefits) was estimated to range from $4,000 to $6,000 (1980$) and research indicated that, after adjusting for differences in time and location, the development costs of a typical public housing unit had been 40 percent higher than unsubsidized construction (Schnare et al., 1982).

2. Many of the previously built publicly assisted projects had become financially distressed — in many cases HUD had to take over management and provide additional funding to bail them out.
3. The concentration of poverty and its associated problems (e.g., vandalism) in large public projects (mostly in big cities) created strongly negative images for the program as a whole.
4. Limited appropriations coupled with the high cost per unit implied that the number of units constructed under these programs could serve only a small fraction of those eligible for assistance. It is estimated that by 1974 only 1.2 million households (15 percent of those eligible for assistance) were being served.[4] Congress became increasingly concerned with the image of providing generous benefits to a small number while the majority of those in need were not helped at all.

HOUSING POLICY SINCE 1980

The 1980s saw important changes in all three federal housing policy approaches. We begin by reviewing changes that occurred in the nation's housing finance system.

Housing Finance

There were two major themes in housing finance policy during the 1980s. Both were in evidence during the preceding decade, but the Reagan administration gave them additional momentum. The first was deregulation. With rapid inflation and tight monetary policies during the 1970s, long term interest rates grew much more slowly than short term rates. Depositors began to move their funds from thrift institutions (where deposit rates were capped by law) to more competitive investments. The thrifts' portfolios were dominated by older mortgages with fixed rates much below those needed for profitability in the new environment. In the 1970s, the federal government began removing controls. The thrifts were allowed to offer a broader variety of instruments to attract household savings and to originate alternative mortgage instruments (such as adjustable-rate and graduated-payment mortgages) that lessened their risk. The Reagan administration went farther, removing the ceiling on deposit rates as well as other restrictions on the range of investments permissible to the thrifts.

The second theme was the expansion of the secondary mortgage market. The privatization of FNMA and the creation of the Government National Mortgage Association (GNMA) and the Federal Home Loan Mortgage Corporation (FHLMC) had led to the broader acceptance of mortgage backed securities in the 1970s. Aggressive management of these institutions continued this trend in the 1980s, further increasing the supply of funds available for mortgages.

As a result of these trends, housing finance has become more integrated in the broader financial system. A more responsive supply of mortgage funds has clearly been one benefit. But there have been costs, most notably in Savings and Loan failures that devastated much of the industry in the latter part of the decade. Most observers would agree that movement toward deregulation was essential to the industry's survival, but the conventional wisdom now is that it came too fast with too little oversight during the transition. In 1989, Congress was told that the full amount required from the taxpayers to address the thrift crisis would be $159 billion. It now appears that the amount will be more like $200 billion.[5]

Housing Assistance

Given their problems as discussed above, and the new administration's lack of enthusiasm for housing subsidies in general, the Reagan administration drastically cut back the housing production programs and openly endorsed an alternative method of delivering assistance, through two closely related programs: housing vouchers (enacted at the Reagan administration's request) and Section 8 certificates, which were created in 1974. Both are hereafter termed the voucher approach.

With these programs, the beneficiaries select their own apartments from those available in the private rental market. They then pay a part of the total rent for the unit—an amount determined by formula based on their income—and a federal subsidy payment makes up the difference. A key condition, however, is that they must live in an apartment that has passed a housing quality inspection. If an eligible household lives in a substandard unit and wants to stay, repairs have to be made before subsidy payments can start, or they can move to another apartment that already meets the standards. If the household already lives in a standard unit, it can receive payments there automatically. Virtually all poor families who do live in standard housing have to pay an unreasonably large share of their income for rent. In such cases, the voucher payments do not change their housing conditions but only ease the pressure on other components of the family budget.

The voucher approach had been tested in a series of major experiments in the 1970s (See Struyk and Bendick, 1981; Kennedy, 1980 and Lowry, 1983). The experiments showed that use of vouchers: (1) did not cause rent inflation (as some had previously feared); (2) had little effect on mobility patterns or neighborhood change; (3) were much less expensive than the production programs; (4) significantly reduced budgetary strains for households that had to pay an excessively large share of their incomes for rent; and (5) had a positive, but only modest effect, on housing quality.

Since vouchers did not have much impact on the supply side, one might have expected little support from housing advocates for the voucher approach. In the late 1970s, however, there was a growing recognition that supply and quality issues were no longer the main determinants of the nation's housing problem. Between 1940 and 1980, the number of occupied housing units in America increased from 34.9 million to 80.4 million. Local housing standards were more rigorously enforced. Deficient units were demolished and replaced by new units of higher quality. The total number of seriously substandard units declined dramatically. For example, only 3 percent of occupied housing units lacked some or all plumbing facilities in 1980, down from 55 percent in 1940.

Over the same period, house prices had accelerated. By the early 1980s, it had become much more difficult for young families to afford to purchase a home (in significant part because of decontrol of mortgage financing). By the late 1980s, renters were having to pay a much larger share of their incomes for rent. In 1983, quality problems still existed but affordability problems were already dominant. Housing problems of all types were much more serious for Very Low Income (VLI) renters (those with incomes below half of medians in their localities):

- 9 percent of all households (but 19 percent of VLI renters) lived in an inadequate unit (as determined by housing quality standards normally used by HUD) (Simonson, 1981).
- 3 percent of all households (but 5 percent of VLI renters) who were not in inadequate units lived in overcrowded conditions (here defined as more than one person per room).
- 17 percent of all households (but 56 percent of VLI renters) not in either of the above categories, had unreasonable cost burdens: i.e., annual housing expenses exceeded 30 percent of incomes (40 percent for homeowners paying into mortgage principal) (Irby, 1983).

In these circumstances, housing vouchers (which cost less and had a direct impact on affordability) appeared a more attractive solution even without an impressive supply effect. Section 8 certificates had been introduced in the late 1970s, but production programs remained dominant during the decade. Over fiscal years (FY) 1977-1980, assistance was provided to an additional 290,000 households per year on average, but 64 percent of them were for the production programs (see Table 1). Under the Reagan administration, the total size of the net addition declined and the emphasis was reversed. Over the FY1982-86 period, the annual net addition in the number of households assisted averaged 79,800, and 84 percent of them were assisted through vouchers and Section 8 certificates. While the voucher programs markedly increased their share in the Reagan years, their net addition had actually declined in absolute terms (from 104,400 annually over 1977-80 to 67,100 annually over 1982-86). Bush administration requests are somewhat higher in total than those for the Reagan

TABLE 1

ADDITIONAL HOUSEHOLDS RECEIVING HUD RENTAL ASSISTANCE
BY PROGRAM TYPE, 1977-1990 (in thousands)

Fiscal Year	Total	Production Programs	Voucher Approach
1977	354.4	226.8	127.6
1978	317.0	190.5	126.5
1979	303.1	200.3	102.8
1980	187.9	129.5	58.4
1981	158.9	75.3	83.6
1982	55.8	17.4	38.4
1983	53.7	6.3	47.4
1984	88.3	9.6	78.7
1985	102.7	16.9	85.8
1986	98.6	13.1	85.5
1987	93.0	20.2	72.8
1988	85.3	20.0	65.3
1989*	94.7	15.6	79.1
1990*	113.4	5.6	107.8

SOURCE: Congressional Budget Office data.
* = Administration request. "Production Programs include Public Housing and Section 8 New Construction and Substantial Rehabilitation. "Voucher Approach" includes Vouchers, and Section 8 Existing Housing and Moderate Rehabilitation programs.

years, and they propose an even higher percentage allocation for the voucher approach.

Since the production programs cost more and require an up front commitment for a much longer period of time, these shifts have implied a precipitous decline in budget authority appropriated (from a high of $29.4 billion in FY1978 to a low of $3.3 billion in 1990 in constant FY1977 dollars).

Still, the number of housing program beneficiaries has continued to grow. The Congressional Budget Office (1988) indicated that at the end of FY1987, 4.30 million households were receiving HUD rental assistance and that sufficient funds had been appropriated to support 4.65 million by the end of FY1988. That number would probably serve 34 percent of the estimated number of eligibles—indeed an impressive change from the 15 percent in 1974 noted earlier.

Tax Incentives

Congress had enacted a number of additional tax benefits for housing during the 1960s and 1970s, but as that period drew to a close, critics argued the trend had gone too far. They suggested that those incentives were inducing overinvestment in housing at the expense of more productive sectors of the economy. The 1986 tax reform (along with other reform legislation passed earlier in the decade) eliminated many of the special benefits for rental housing. These were replaced with a new Low Income Housing Tax Credit (LIHTC), under which most of the subsidized new construction of housing for the poor was carried out in 1988 and 1989.

With the reduction in marginal tax rates, even those features that were not touched (most important, the deductibility of mortgage interest payments) lost much of their potency as investment incentives.

Even so, the housing tax losses that remain have tremendous budgetary impact. The three largest in the Bush Administration's FY1991 budget are: (1) deductibility of homeowner mortgage interest—$46.6 billion; (2) rollover of capital gains when homes are sold—$13.3 billion; (3) homeowner deductions for local property tax payments—$12.4 billion. Together, these account for tax expenditures of $72.3 billion, most of which benefit middle- and upper-income groups. In contrast, the total budget authority appropriated for HUD housing programs for FY 1990 was $13.1 billion.

FUTURE POLICIES

In this section we look forward to policy and other developments in the housing sector likely in the years immediately ahead, based in part on the trends just reviewed. Broad developments are briefly considered first, and then we turn more specifically to the elderly.

Overall Policy Trends

Developments in *housing finance* will be driven by demographics and the continuing effects of the S&L crisis. The sharp decline in the rate of household formations associated with the baby bust will produce a decline in mortgage originations generally. At the same time, however, the volume of loans going to secondary markets may remain constant or even increase, because of the risk-based capital requirements of the Financial Institutions Reform, Recovery, and Enforcement Act (FIRREA)—the S&L rescue legislation. In particular, FIRREA requires different capital amounts for different types of assets, depending on their riskiness. Mortgages have a higher capital requirement than mortgaged-backed securities, for example; so S&Ls will be selling more of the mortgages they originate in secondary markets.

FIRREA increases the overall level of capital required of thrift institutions (as a percent of assets) as well as differentiating among various assets. For this reason, among others, a continuing shakeout in the thrift industry is expected over the next several years, with perhaps one-third of all S&Ls disappearing. One consequence will be a greater role in mortgage origination by commercial banks and mortgage bankers. Even with all of these changes, however, mortgage funds should remain plentiful, although their cost relative to those on other debt may rise somewhat because of the more stringent capital requirements.

Changes in *housing assistance policy* are also expected. While the relative emphasis on housing vouchers (versus new construction programs) will continue, the Bush Administration is proposing a clear shift to using housing as a tool to address problems of persistent poverty. Its FY1991 budget proposals place heavy emphasis on homeownership for very low income families, converting public housing and other projects already serving the poor to owner-occupancy. The belief is that changing renters with little control over their lives into homeowners will increase the new homeowners' motivation to work, to send their children to school, and to take charge of their lives more generally.

The same theme of combining support services and housing assistance to help families "break out" of their current circumstances is repeated elsewhere in the FY1991 proposals. In the future, localities would have to have a program for helping those able-bodied unemployed persons receiving housing assistance with training and other programs to increase their employability. Similar provisions apply to some of the help to be provided to the homeless.

The Congress has not rejected these proposals out of hand and hence they may mark a turning point in the orientation of housing assistance. The Administration's proposals, as well as omnibus housing bills introduced in both the House and Senate in 1989, also call for greater contributions from the states for housing assistance. On the other hand, while the Congressional proposals have pressed for greater federal funding for housing assistance, the Bush budget proposals, when carefully adjusted for renewing expiring contracts and other factors, leave levels essentially unchanged in nominal dollars from the previous year. This, too, may be a continuing phenomenon.

Finally, *tax expenditures* for housing may change in the years ahead, but developments here are much harder to read. A key factor is that under Gramm-Rudman pressures, tax expenditures are soon likely to be allocated by functional budget categories in the same way budget authority is: the days of "extra spending" through taxes may be numbered. In this context, assistance for low-income housing via taxes, as through the Low Income Housing Tax Credit, may vanish, with the equivalent budget authority being transferred to the authorizing and appropriations committees. A more speculative possible development might come from continued growth in homeownership tax expenditures. Granted, the baby bust should cut the growth rate of these expenditures, but if, under the evolving rules of accounting for such expenditures in the federal budget, they begin to impinge on housing assistance levels, there *could* be pressure to contain them in some form. Given the popularity of these provisions, however, the chances for meaningful reductions seem remote.

All in all, then, there may be some important legislative changes over the next year or so, but there is nothing on the horizon to indicate any fundamental change in U.S. housing policy from that established in the Reagan years. Housing assistance may be more tightly focused on the poor and delivered in new ways to support their empowerment and access to needed services. States and localities may be made the dominant actors as far as production assistance is concerned. But neither budget increases big enough to significantly increase the percent of eligible households being served nor major reductions in tax expenditures benefitting middle-income homeowners seem to be in the cards in the short term.

Housing problems are likely to remain in the limelight, however, so we can expect continuing pressure for more substantial change in the years to come. Two forces will keep the topic alive. First is dearth of affordable housing. Largely due to rigid local regulations, modestly priced housing continues to decline as a share of the total stock and, given increasing poverty, this implies that the problem of homelessness is almost sure to expand. Second is the tremendous demographic change underway in American society. Traditional two parent families are rapidly declining as a proportion of all households while other groups (the elderly and non-elderly single parents and single individuals living alone or in groups) are experiencing enormous growth.[6] These new households typically require less space and have different physical and locational requirements than the traditional families for which most of our existing housing stock was built. The stock changes slowly. There will be sizeable frictions and frustrations in adapting it to meet changing requirements.

Future Housing Policy for the Elderly

For analytic purposes it is useful to divide the housing problems of the elderly into two groups. One group consists of the "traditional" housing problems — occupancy of deficient units and spending an excessive share of income on housing.[7] The second is the difficulty experienced by the frail elderly in continuing to live independently in their own homes or apartments and the responses to these difficulties in the form of unit modification or provision of support services.

With respect to the traditional housing problems, until recently the poor elderly could be cited as a disadvantaged group, i.e., having a higher incidence of these problems than their nonelderly counterparts. This is no longer the case: through a combination of very substantial growth in incomes of the elderly over the past two decades and higher than proportional participation in government assistance programs by elderly renters, the poor elderly now closely resemble the rest of the poverty population in this regard. In the future, advocates of the elderly can argue for the elderly receiving their "fair share" of the available resources, but they cannot claim a special level of need.

The frail elderly are another story. Federal housing assistance has all but neglected this group. The only integrated package of housing and support services explicitly targeted to the frail elderly is the very small Congregate Housing Services Program (CHSP). Importantly, the Administration has not recommended and the Congress has not acted to dedicate housing projects specially designed for elderly occupancy for the frail elderly. While many of these projects do serve frail persons (as do projects without special features), the targeting of available assistance on the frail elderly is currently quite weak overall.

There are signs, however, that both the Congress and Administration are beginning to explore ways to provide integrated packages of housing and support services to the frail elderly. As part of the Housing and Community Development Act of 1987, Congress mandated that HUD do a study of options in this area. The Bush Administration introduced a new model for providing a housing-services package to frail elderly already receiving housing assistance (either project- or tenant-based) as part of its FY1991 budget submission to Congress based on the options developed in the study (see below).[8] And all of the omnibus housing bills recently introduced in Congress make some further provision for creating such packages.

The next few years are likely to see a moderate degree of experimentation with alternative models for providing the housing-services package in order to find the most cost-effective option. Cost-effectiveness is a critical issue within the Administration and among many in Congress because of the widespread view that the country cannot afford to take on another expensive social program. The key to expanding federal support for housing-services packages for lower income families is to demonstrate that their costs are largely, if not fully, offset by savings to Medicaid, Medicare, and locally funded support service programs. To date, the CHSP has not been able to demonstrate such savings. The report prepared in response to the Congressional mandate reaches some important conclusions about the design of future programs based on the experience of the CHSP and similar programs operated by the states.[9]

First, in selecting the elderly to receive supportive services, those evaluating prospective participants must be trained and given clear guidance on the degree of impairment that constitutes sufficient severity to warrant admission. Given current knowledge, a reasonable standard that could be implemented consistently is the presence of at least one activity of daily living limitation severe enough to require personal assistance and one or more instrumental activity of daily living limitation. Use of a centralized screening system at the local level, rather than staff at each project conducting their own assessments, is preferable because it permits more consistent application of guidelines in a process that inevitably requires judgments to be made.

Careful case management and tailoring of services are central to any cost containment effort and to effectively meeting the individual needs of participants. The skills of the on-site coordinator and regular contact with the coordinator, as at mealtimes, are important in this regard. Formal client evaluation and modification of the service package should be repeated at least annually after admission into the program. Moreover, co-payments from participants, based on income and on the quantity of services received, are advisable, both to offset program costs and to help contain service use.

A core package of nonmedical services should be offered at each facility, but mandatory participation in a service is justifiable only when economies of scale in its provision outweigh tailoring considerations, as may be so with congregate meal service. A higher level of services (including medical services) than can be offered by congregate programs could be arranged through state Medicaid offices using waivered home and community-based service options.

In terms of tailoring and avoidance of overservicing, there are strong arguments for providing cash payments to housing providers with which to purchase services from vendors or to deliver them directly, rather than forcing projects to broker in-kind services from several sources that are funded directly by a variety of state agencies. Unifying the sources of funds to the provider into a single payment would simplify management and coordination tasks. In the case of federally assisted housing, channeling the funds through a single federal agency is appropriate. These changes would leave coordinators freer to fit services specifically to client needs and to provide needed services themselves, where appropriate, or to purchase them from vendors offering a less expensive quality product.

Although programs currently operating could be — and in many cases are being — modified to be consistent with the lessons learned from experience to date, most have a substantial distance to go. Several possible new approaches show promise for serving frail elderly residents of assisted housing. They include the Housing and Support Services Certificate Program, social/health maintenance organizations, and the Congregate Housing Certificate Program.

Under the Housing Support Services Certificate Program (HSSCP), frail elders determined by the administering agent (the local housing authority or a nonprofit organization, possibly including a current sponsor in the Section 202 program) to be eligible would receive a certificate covering the costs of support services. The payments for services would be used by the local administering agent to provide case management and the necessary support services, either directly or through various vendors. In principle, the agent could contract out the whole case management and service delivery responsibility; it could also contract with several vendors and allow households to select among them. HSSCP has yet to be implemented, but it is the model proposed by the Bush Administration in its FY1991 budget submission.

Four social/health maintenance organizations (S/HMOs) have been in operation on a demonstration basis since 1985. Under this model, a single private provider organization assumes responsibility for a full range of ambulatory, acute inpatient, nursing home, home health, and personal care services under a prospectively determined fixed budget. All elderly residents of assisted housing in a locality would be encouraged to enroll in an S/HMO that would then be wholly responsible for case management, tailoring, and provision of services to clients. The residents' monthly capitated enrollment fees would be subsidized in whole or in part.

Under the Congregate Housing Certificate Program (CHCP), which exists only in concept, households eligible on the basis of low income and high risk of institutionalization would receive a certificate entitling them to occupy a unit in a congregate housing project that provides independent living with the necessary nonmedical support services. The voucher would cover the cost of both housing and the level of support services warranted, with the households contributing 50-60 percent of their incomes toward the combined costs. As proposed, vouchers could be used at approved privately operated facilities.

These options represent several of many that could be developed from basic building blocks designed to improve targeting, control costs, and improve tailoring of services to match needs. The amount of responsibility assigned to agencies versus that given to individual elderly persons for securing services, the extent of integration of payments for housing and support services, and the application of and approach to existing housing programs could all be varied. The models presented are good examples of what could be done.

These promising options should be further developed and evaluated. Now is an appropriate time for experimentation among these options in light of the growing population of frail elderly and the uncertainty about how best to proceed. Such experimentation seems likely in the years ahead, given the policy proposals tabled by the Administration and the Congress in early 1990 and the fact that such experimentation will make very modest demands on the federal budget.

ENDNOTES

1. For full discussions of the evolutions of America's housing finance system, during this period and thereafter, see Tucillo, 1973, and Hendershott and Villani, 1977.

2. These data are calculated from the Bureau of the Census (1975) series which shows the total stock of low rent public housing under management (occupied or available for occupancy) increasing from 201,700 units in 1950 to 478,200 units in 1960 and 893,500 units in 1970.

3. More complete examinations of the history of these programs are provided in Struyk et al., 1983, and Struyk et al., 1988.

4. Burke (1984) estimated that there were 8.4 million very low income renter households in 1974, out of which 1.2 million were receiving HUD subsidies. The number of very low income renter households (those with incomes at or below 50 percent of the median incomes in their communities) is usually considered equivalent to the total number of eligibles.

5. David Rosenbaum, New York Times 3/18/90.

6. See the more complete discussion of these trends and their implications for housing policy in Struyk, Turner, and Ueno, 1988.

7. A third problem — overcrowding — is usually included in this group. However, this has not been a problem for the elderly in the past and certainly is not currently.

8. The same package, however, also provided no funding for continuing or expanding the CHSP. Prior Administrations have made the same proposal but have been turned back by the Congress.

9. Struyk, Page, Newman et al. (1989).

REFERENCES

Bureau of the Census (1975). *Historical Statistics of the United States: Colonial Times to 1970,* U.S. Department of Commerce, Washington.

―――― (1982), *Annual Housing Survey, 1980, Part A: General Housing Characteristics,* U.S. Department of Commerce, Washington.

Burke, Paul (1984), "Trends in Subsidized Housing, 1974-81," unpublished paper, Division of Housing and Demographic Analysis, Office of Economic Affairs, U.S. Department of Housing and Urban Development, Washington.

Congressional Budget Office (1988), *Current Housing Problems and Possible Federal Responses,* Congress of the United States, Washington.

Downs, A. (1988). A Strategy for Designing a Fully Comprehensive National Housing Policy for the Federal Government of the United States. Washington, D.C.: U.S. Government Printing Office p. 2.

Irby, Iredia (1986), "Attaining the Housing Goal?," unpublished paper, Division of Housing and Demographic Analysis, Office of Economic Affairs, U.S. Department of Housing and Urban Development, Washington.

Kennedy, Stephen D. (1980) "Final Report of the Housing Allowance Demand Experience." Submitted to the Office of Policy Development and Research, U.S. Department of Housing and Urban Development, Washington, D.C. Cambridge, MA: Abt Associates.

Lowry, Ira S. ed. (1983), *Experimenting with Housing Allowances: The Final Report of the Housing Assistance Supply Experiment,* Oeleschlager, Gunn and Hain, Cambridge.

Mayo et al. (1980), *Housing Allowances and Other Housing Assistance Programs — A Comparison Based on the Housing Allowance Demand Experiment, Part 2: Cost and Efficiency,* Abt Associates, Inc., Cambridge.

Schnare, Ann B., et al. (1982), *The Costs of HUD Multifamily Programs,* Urban

Systems Research and Engineering, U.S. Department of Housing and Urban Development, Washington.

Simonson, J. (1981), *Measuring Inadequate Housing Through Use of the Annual Housing Survey,* U.S. Department of Housing and Urban Development, Office of Policy Development and Research, Washington.

Struyk, Raymond J., and Marc Bendick, Jr. (1981), *Housing Vouchers for the Poor: Lessons from a National Experiment,* Urban Institute Press, Washington.

Struyk, Raymond J., Neil Mayer, and John A. Tuccillo (1983), *Federal Housing Policy at President Reagan's Midterm,* Urban Institute, Wwashington.

Struyk, Raymond J., Margery A. Turner, and Makiko Ueno (1988), *Future U.S. Housing Policy,* The Urban Institute Press, Washington.

Tuccillo, John A., with John L. Goodman (1983), *Housing Finance: A Changing System in the Reagan Era,* Urban Institute Press, Washington.

Assessing Consumer Need and Demand for Service-Assisted Housing in Pennsylvania

Barbara Granger
Lenard W. Kaye

INTRODUCTION

State level concern in Pennsylvania's Governor's Office and Department of Aging about housing options for middle income older people has been growing in recent years. This concern led recently to a request for a statewide survey. The purpose of the survey was to assess the need for service assisted housing (SAH) in Pennsylvania and gauge preferences for different service assisted housing options.

Service assisted housing is a relatively new approach in meeting the need for housing options for middle income older people. The Pennsylvania Department on Aging (PDA) defines SAH as housing which is:

- for persons 60 + who are independent and healthy
- a self-contained apartment in a multi-unit complex
- a moderately priced rental apartment
- available without an entrance fee

Barbara Granger, MCP, is Research Associate at Matrix Research Institute, a non-profit research and training center in Philadelphia. Ms. Granger has used research as a tool for policy, planning, evaluation, community development and advocacy activities — all of which have been directed at assisting organizations in creating alternative supportive communities and innovative services. She has taught social policy, social theory and community organization practice courses at Temple University, Antioch College and Bryn Mawr College. Lenard W. Kaye, DSW, is Professor and Associate Dean at the Bryn Mawr College Graduate School of Social Work and Social Research in Bryn Mawr, PA.

This research was funded by the Pennsylvania Department of Aging, Contract No. 887003.

- an apartment complex not attached to a continuum of care
- linked to flexible levels of supportive services, personal care and minimal health services which are: (1) provided only as needed and on a fee-for-service basis, and (2) coordinated through the housing provider (PDA, 1988).

In 1988, PDA sponsored an internal study to explore the need for and availability of SAH in the Commonwealth. Based on demographic analysis, they estimated that 87,398 Pennsylvania elderly could benefit from this housing option. Their recommendations included the need for a comprehensive statewide survey of a representative sample of older persons assessing their need for and interest in SAH. Findings from this survey, which are reported in this article, suggest that there exists an even greater potential market for this type of housing—23% of older people over age 60 would be interested in SAH. Based on a 1988 Pennsylvania population figure of 2,384,000 persons over age 60, estimated SAH interest could be as high as 548,320. Despite differences in the comparative methodologies of the 1988 PDA study and the analysis reported here, substantial numbers of older people in Pennsylvania appear to be in need of and interested in service assisted housing options.

LITERATURE REVIEW

Affordable and adequate housing has become increasingly a rare commodity for Americans. This is especially true for many older people with fixed incomes who face escalating housing and maintenance costs. Declining health, retirement from the workplace, loss of a spouse or significant friends, fear of crime, displacement due to condominium conversion, and job mobility of offspring frequently can result in growing isolation and loneliness for older persons. Without adequate support services in the community, these factors may contribute to individuals' becoming more physically, socially, and financially vulnerable than is warranted. This vulnerability oftentimes results in premature or unnecessary institutionalization. Although there are other options that combine housing and support services, such as continuing care retirement communities, congregate housing programs, shared living homes, and personal care homes (Tiven & Ryther, 1986), each with its own unique character and development requirements, service assisted housing is specifically designed for moderate income older persons who cannot afford large entrance fees, yet earn too much income for subsidized rental units. A combination of rental housing and appropriate services for this population is scarce at present.

Housing developers are likely to respond to this need only if they can be sufficiently assured that older persons will choose (or demand) the service assisted housing option. Several demographic and social trends — reviewed below — suggest that they will.

The housing market for older people is likely to experience dramatic changes over the next few decades, dictated by current and projected demographic imperatives. The percentage of older people in the United States has almost tripled since 1900 to roughly 12% of the total population, or 26 million people. This number is expected to increase to 20% (or 59 million persons) when the postwar baby boom cohort reaches retirement (Davis, 1983). Older Pennsylvanians currently conform to this national projection. Older persons were expected to comprise 19% of Pennsylvania's total population in 1990, and 24% of the population by 2030 (PDA, 1983).

In addition to the increasing numbers of older persons, however, several other factors influence a demand for service assisted housing. These include (1) increases in the proportion of older women; (2) an increase in the proportion of homeowners; (3) the uneven migration patterns of older persons who are relocating; and (4) special housing needs for widows living alone as well as for minorities (Newman, 1985; Longino, 1979; AARP, 1989). According to Lawton and Hoover (1981), older suburban residents are of particular interest; the growth rate of this group was almost three times that of the older population in central cities, and they would appear candidates for SAH options.

Finally, service assisted housing, which provides housing-related services such as housekeeping, meals, and social activities, attempts to meet needs traditionally addressed informally through family, friend and neighbor networks. Research confirms, however, that the increase of dual income, mobile families has served to diminish the availability of such support (Brody, 1981). For instance, resident managers of existing rental housing programs for the elderly reported at an October, 1988 conference (Federation Housing, Inc.) that family and friends are not always available as often as they are needed. Service assisted housing can be designed to provide for supportive services to meet the needs of middle income older persons. Middle income older people can afford to purchase a fuller complement of services than those offered in government subsidized housing, while they are not usually able to afford the more expensive luxury rental housing or continuing care retirement communities.

The wide array of demographic and social factors reviewed above appear to converge in such a way as to make SAH a viable option. But is it really an affordable and attractive alternative for older persons? It should be underscored here that one of the consistent themes of this assessment research is the distinction that must be made between the *need* for SAH options and the likely demand for such services. Need estimates provide, in this instance, a broad assessment of the numbers of moderate income elderly persons who could conceivably make use of affordable rental housing in conjunction with special services. The 1988 Pennsylvania Department of Aging-sponsored internal SAH report indeed estimates considerable need for SAH in Pennsylvania. However, it is the ability to project demand for, or actual interest in, the SAH option among all those elderly persons who could conceivably need service assisted housing that assists in housing development decisions. That is, housing developers are interested in the extent to which older people are more likely than not to choose and pay for an SAH option.

METHODOLOGY

The methodology for this research included the combination of a statewide structured mail survey of older people, key informant interviews and the performance of four focus group sessions. The primary source of data for this report is the statewide survey.

Survey Sample

The Pennsylvania Department of Transportation provided a random sampling of 1500 individuals over the age of 60 from their listing of licensed drivers. They were instructed to over-sample women to reflect the current male/female ratio in the state. The ratio of 40.9% men and 59.1% women is based on the Pennsylvania State Data Center's population estimates for July 1, 1985 and 1986. There were a total of 597 (40%) returns from the initial mailing and follow-up reminder to the 1500 older licensed drivers. After eliminating inappropriate responses, the mailing yielded a final respondent sample of 586 codeable surveys.

The respondent group compares favorably to the older resident population in the Commonwealth on a series of demographic profile variables. Regional comparisons across population and respondent data sets indicate a slightly higher survey response realized from the southeast and southwest regions which are the more urbanized areas of the state and lower responses from the northwest and northeast regions. The mean age for both the original random sample and the respondent survey sample is 69 years with comparable age concentrations spread across age range categories. The original random sample was comprised of 58% women and 42% men, while the survey respondents were made up of 60% women and 40% men. As might be expected, more responding men (83%) are married than women (55%); while more responding women (33%) are widowed than men (9%). These figures are comparable to nationwide statistics reported by AARP (1988).

The educational level for older people nationally and the respondent sample both show that almost half have completed high school or trade school; however, the respondent sample is more likely to be college educated (17%) than those nationwide (10%) (AARP, 1988). A slightly greater proportion of the survey sample (16%) are employed than are elders nationally (11%); however, respondent income data are comparable to national figures, with two-thirds of the former reporting household income under $20,000 per year (AARP, 1988).

In the Health Profile of Older Pennsylvanians (1988) almost two-thirds of older people (60%) rate their health as "good" or "very good." Survey respondents report a somewhat higher rate of "good" or "very good" health (77%), indicating that health problems cause less difficulties for licensed older drivers managing their household than elder residents in general. However, over 90% of both groups report having no difficulties with everyday activities.

Home ownership rates for the respondent sample and elders nationally (AARP, 1988) are comparable (87% and 85% respectively), and almost one-third of both report that they live alone (27% and 30% respectively). With few exceptions, respondent data reported here are comparable to those reported for the earlier Pennsylvania and related national studies.

Study Variables

The mailed survey was structured to include questions related to older persons' current housing situation, overall housing preferences, preferences for SAH options (design, costs, services and amenities), interest in SAH, and overall demographic characteristics. The survey questions were primarily forced-choice questions with several open-ended questions to gauge the reasons behind particular choices and opinions. The survey was reviewed by a Project Advisory Committee made up of experienced professionals engaged in aging and housing-related research and program development activities and pre-tested prior to mailing.

The dependent variable in this study is "interest in the service assisted housing option." A second set of independent variables which are believed to potentially influence choice include attitudinal characteristics reflecting the personal preferences, motivations and perceptions concerning this housing option.

Interviews

Further data concerning factors which would influence interest in SAH were collected through: (1) 18 key informant interviews; and (2) 4 focus group sessions. Individual interviews were conducted with 7 developers, 5 development consultants and 6 SAH-type residence managers. Key informants were identified by members of the Project Advisory Committee, newspaper advertisements, and presenters at a recent national retirement housing conference. The focus group interviews were conducted in three different regions of the state and were carried out with four different sets of people: housing developers, gerontological practitioners, elder family members and older residents from an SAH development. Analysis of data focused on the identification of (1) categories of information or issues, and (2) key questions for developers or SAH consumers.

FINDINGS

Selected results of the analysis are summarized in Table 1. The profile provides a comparative overview of those who are and those who are not interested in SAH. From the outset, findings indicate that basic descriptive information (i.e., age, sex, marital status, health status, education and income) reflects no differences between the two groups with the exception of whether or not one rents or owns their current housing. Overall, survey respondents report that most (75%) are "satisfied" with their current housing, while 25% are "less than satisfied" or "dissatisfied" with their homes. Survey respondents report that "problems with home maintenance" (67%) and "one's own poor health" (56%) are the primary reasons for wanting to move. However, interest in possessions (54%) is the primary reason for postponing moving. Some respondents (22%) have considered moving in the past two years, most of these (18%) to apartments. However, when asked specifically about an SAH apartment choice, 23% of respondents indicated interest in moving to an SAH apartment now, and 39% would do so in the future.

SAH Physical Design

Based on first stage analysis and a series of chi squares, no significant differences were found concerning preferences in SAH physical or service design between respondents who were or were not interested in SAH. Consequently, findings are aggregated when reporting SAH design data.

Almost half of the respondents expect to live alone (48%), with half of these (23%) preferring a one bedroom apartment, 19% a two bedroom, and 6% a studio/efficiency apartment. The other half of the respondents (48%) expect to live with another person and most (41%) want a two bedroom, with 7% preferring a one bedroom, apartment. Taken together, 6% prefer a studio, 30% a one bedroom, and 61% a two bedroom apartment (3% were undecided).

Almost half (45%) expect to pay rent of less than $300 per month, with 32% willing to pay to $400, 12% up to $500, and 11% over $500 per month. Most (66%) prefer a low rise building, but 29% would be satisfied with either a high-rise or low-rise building. Almost three-quarters of respondents prefer an SAH be located outside the city, in the suburbs (37%) or a small town (36%).

SAH Service Design

These preferences are also based on the full respondent sample, as there were no significant differences between SAH interest groups. SAH is characterized by its provision of supportive services and specialized amenities. Respondents report their strongest interest (71%) in heavy housecleaning services, additional interest in light housekeeping services (63%) and one meal per day (60%), and less interest in two meals per day (49%). In all cases, respondents preferred to pay for services separately, rather than as part of their rent.

In addition to rent, a little over half (57%) of respondents would pay $100 per month or less for these services, 28% would pay up to $200, 6% up to $300, and 9% over $300.

Respondents also provided their preferences for other services that they would like to be available for their use. The top four services of interest to our respondents are availability of a grocery store (91%), doctors' offices (88%), a pharmacy (82%), and a beauty/barbershop (71%). There was less interest expressed in a dry cleaner (54%), nursing services (50%), home care services (44%), or a gift shop (36%). In all cases, more respondents preferred these services to be available near the SAH, rather than on-site.

Respondents reported the following leisure activities of interest. Most respondents want walking paths (76%) on-site (71%), religious services (69%) near the SAH (58%), and a library (58%) on-site (59%). Almost half the respondents were interested in having a social/recreational staff (47%) on-site (77%), and a swimming pool (46%) on-site (74%), with somewhat less interest in cultural programming (44%), garden space (39%), shuffleboard/ horseshoes (25%), or tennis courts (11%).

Most (85%) respondents feel it is important to have security personnel in the apartment building and 93% want an emergency call button in the apartment. Most respondents (88%) own a car and almost all (98%) will need a parking space. (This finding must be considered in light of the sample having been drawn from licensed drivers.) However, almost half (43%) are interested in using an apartment van and over half (53%) are interested in using public transportation. There are no significant differences in the relative strength of individual preferences for any of the leisure services and amenities listed in Table 6 when comparing those who are interested in the SAH option and those who are not.

Correlational Analysis

Further analysis explores the strength of relationships among a wide variety of study variables. Table 2 presents the correlation coefficients for a series of demographic and attitudinal study variables. As shown, significant correlations cluster around the attitudinal variables and interest in SAH rather than the demographic variables. To examine the relative contribution of each variable, least squares regression analysis was used with "interest in service assisted housing" serving as the outcome or dependent variable. Using the stepwise entry method for the eleven variables, entering the equation at PIN.10 and POUT.10 levels of specification, 32% of the variance is explained. Table 3 summarizes the regression data. The most influential predictor variable is the attitudinal variable of "one's interest in SAH as a housing option while still healthy and independent." It should be noted that only the first five variables are significant predictors at the $p < .05$ level, representing 28% of the explained variance; while the remaining six variables, primarily demographic factors, contribute little to the overall explanation and do not meet customary significance requirements.

TABLE 1. Profile Comparison of Consumers Interested in Service Assisted Housing and Those Not Interested

	Interested In SAH (n=122)	Not Interested In SAH (n=182)	Significance
	Percentage	Percentage	
Age			
60-69	63	63	t = 0.06, n.s.
70-79	29	30	
80+	8	7	
Sex			
Women	38	39	$\chi^2 = 0.07$, n.s.
Men	62	61	
Marital Status			
Married	62	72	$\chi^2 = 4.70$, n.s.
Not Married (single, widowed, divorced, or separated)	38	27	
Housing			
Rent	26	4	$\chi^2 = 33.86$ (p > .001)
Private Home	73	94	
Health Status			
Problems	29	19	$\chi^2 = 4.26$, n.s.
No Problems	70	81	
Education			
Some grade school	3	2	t = -1.78, n.s.
Grade school complete	4	10	
Some high school	14	8	
High school complete	43	34	
Business or trade school	7	8	
Some college	16	14	
College complete	9	11	
Graduate School	3	12	
Income			
$0 - $19,999	56	40	$\chi^2 = 1.52$, n.s.
$20,000 or more	37	46	
Missing Data	7	14	

TABLE 2. Correlations for Selected Demographic and Attitudinal Variables

	SAHAVAIL	SAHINDP	SAHTRBL	HOMPMT	AGERES
SAHAVAIL	1.0000				
SAHINDP	.4292**	1.0000			
SAHTRBL	-.1590*	.0121	1.0000		
HOMPMT	-.2689**	-.1295	-.0050	1.0000	
AGERES	-.1411*	-.0749	-.0318	.0053	1.0000
EDUC	-.1007	-.1314	.0096	.0424	-.0588
SATHOM	-.2358**	-.2287**	.0844	.0428*	-.0125
LOCHOM	.1281	-.0723	-.1074	-.0833	-.0420
SEX	-.0489	-.0034	.0410	-.0233	.1817*
HHNORES	-.0811	-.0666	-.0671	.0944	.0541
AGE	-.0430	.0603	.0479	-.1121	-.0466
INCOME	-.0663	-.1152	-.0513	.1333	-.0716

SAHAVAIL - interest in service assisted housing

SAHINDP - interest in SAH while still healthy and independent

SAHTRBL - interest in SAH only if having trouble maintaining own home

HOMPMT   - consumer as renter or home owner

AGERES   - preference for age of SAH residents

DISCUSSION

Health and Independence

An important finding emerging from this analysis is the rationale behind choosing an SAH. Those who would want to move into an SAH now want to do so while still able-bodied, independent, and able to maintain their own residence. Those who are not interested in an SAH would expect to choose an SAH only if they have trouble maintaining their own home, or if poor health or loss of independence required it. That is to say, those interested in SAH perceive it more as a housing option; while those not interested in SAH value it more for its supportive services.

More (32%) of those interested in SAH live alone than those not interested in SAH (22%). In addition, despite interest in SAH while still

EDUC	SATHOM	LOCHOM	SEX	HHNORES	AGE	INCOME
1.0000						
.0491	1.0000					
.1545*	-.0212	1.0000				
-.0622	-.0197	-.0204	1.0000			
-.0074	.0224	.1082	-.0977	1.0000		
-.0314	.0204	-.0726	-.1182	-.1492*	1.0000	
.3063**	.0411	.1566*	-.1322	.1234	-.1031	

```
EDUC     - education
SATHON   - satisfaction with current home
LOCHOM   - location of home--urban, suburban, small town, country
HHNORES  - number of residents in current household
( * = p< .001 and ** = p<.001)
```

healthy and independent, more (29%) of those interested in SAH report that health problems cause them some difficulties at home than those (19%) not interested. However, both groups indicate a high level of functional capacity in carrying out everyday activities.

While the average age of the respondents is 69 years, key informants who were interviewed (i.e., housing developers) report that the average age of applicants to SAH-type apartments is 75 years. In six years, our survey respondents' health needs and expectations for supportive services may increase. Key informants report that they found it useful to provide *access* to health care and medical services for temporary use, such as locating medical offices on-site, providing priority access to a related long-term care facility, offering a health plan to SAH residents providing free days at a related facility, having 24-hour on-call nursing services, or making a section of the SAH apartments into a "personal care wing." Furthermore, key informants reported that although an SAH renter may

TABLE 3. Regression of Independent Variables on Interest in Service Assisted Housing (SAH)

Variables	B	Beta	t<p	R Square
Interest in SAH while still healthy and independent	:27	.37	.0000	.18
Rental or Home Owner Status	-.47	-.18	.0009	.04
Interest in SAH if having trouble maintaining own home	-.15	-.16	.002	.03
Location of current home	.22	.13	.013	.02
Attitude about age of other SAH residents	.03	-.11	.028	.01
Satisfaction with current home	-.15	-.10	.06	.01
Education	-.04	-.08	.13	.00
Age	-.07	-.07	.16	.00
Number of residents in current household	-.07	-.07	.19	.00
Sex	-.09	-.05	.35	.00
Income	-.00	-.02	.78	.00

Total R Square = .30

meet the health status application criteria, he or she will "age in place" requiring increasingly more supportive services. Thus, although those interested in SAH report less of a need for basic services currently offered in SAH-type facilities, such services would offer support that could sustain independent living as residents "age in place" (Pynoos, 1988).

Researchers reported in a Pennsylvania study conducted by Hamlym Associates (1989) that older people (average age 75 to 79 years) who live in low income, subsidized congregate housing projects want and need supportive services available to them. Services of particular interest are assistance with heavy household chores, transportation, assistance with shopping, case management and assistance with light household chores. However, they are unable to pay market rates for these services. Congregate housing (HUD-sponsored) offers group meals, but not other services offered in the SAH model.

Another perspective was offered by participants in a series of focus group interviews with SAH-type residents. We asked how they might respond to someone concerned about losing their independence when moving to an SAH. Their response was immediate and filled with laughter: "that's a fallacy, you gain independence . . . it makes you strong . . . you have freedom to participate in more ways than ever before — lots of activities . . . they're good losses — loss of drudgery . . . no more shopping, cooking, drying dishes, taking out garbage."

Affordability

Since this study is focused on the possibility of private sector SAH development, it is important to discuss affordability. Key informants report that the rent-up process of leasing all apartments in an SAH complex is lengthy, averaging 2.5 units per month for for-profit SAH-type apartments, and 4 units per month for non-profits. This difference is attributed to the not-for-profit's altruistic purposes and more direct access to target consumer groups. However, despite the lengthy initial "rent-up schedule," developers report a very low turnover rate among SAH renters.

Although "satisfaction with current housing" contributes minimally to explaining interest in SAH, there is a significant relationship ($r = -.24$, $p < .001$) between these two variables, indicating that respondents who are dissatisfied with their current housing arrangements are more likely to be interested in an SAH option. Furthermore, it would appear that these individuals may be in a good financial position to afford the SAH option. Survey findings indicate that 71% of those interested in SAH own their own homes and receive regularized income from Social Security (81%), pensions (56%), and investments (47%). In a related study by the Real Estate Research Corporation (RERC) (1986) based on a survey of 42 rental retirement housing projects, researchers report that "the average owner 65 or over has $60,900 in home equity . . . [generating] . . . an additional $470 per month." RERC's report also clarifies perceptions about older people's income. Studies show that rather than living on "fixed incomes," their income tends to be better protected against inflation (especially Social Security) than the income of younger consumers, and that (given retirement status) older people are able to be more frugal.

Furthermore, based on demographics, RERC predicted that for older people aged 75 and over (note that this is the average SAH application age), 35% are able to pay $1,000 per month, 24% could pay $1,200 per month, and 15% could pay $1,500 per month. These predictions were based on a rental retirement option which includes SAH-type support services and on an individual income which includes home equity and other income sources.

Indeed, a cash income comparison between Pennsylvania survey respondents in the study reported here and the RERC national demographic predictions indicates approximately the same proportion of consumers as the national average reporting comparable incomes: survey respondents (age 60 +) in this study who are interested in SAH have an annual income of $20,000-$30,000; the RERC study reports that 15% of those age 65 + have an annual income of $19,500-$32,000. Therefore, despite the fact that survey respondents in this analysis would prefer to pay less for an SAH apartment, the ability to pay actual costs for an affordable SAH for middle income Pennsylvanians is supportable based on both income range and availability of home equity.

Location

Another point of interest to prospective SAH developers is site selection. These survey data suggest another important set of variables to be considered: whether or not a person owns or rents their home and where their home is located. Both key informants and focus group participants report that older people in urban areas are more receptive to the rental housing option, while those in small towns and rural areas tend to identify more strongly with home ownership which appears to be equated with personal identity and independence. Survey data support this conclusion. Respondents who are interested in the SAH option are more likely to be renters and live in urban and suburban areas. Furthermore, it would appear that site selection should include consideration of those services and amenities that older people would prefer to have offered within the SAH and those that can best be provided in the community surrounding the SAH.

Although the data from this study point to influences that may be related to personal attitudes, health status, rental or home ownership status, dissatisfaction with current housing, and location of current housing, one must be careful about making any predictions, given the limited overall contribution of the regression findings. Further research appears warranted that would consider assessing the needs and preferences of older people in relation to their attitudes toward both the segregated and integrated purposes of a housing option with supportive services.

REFERENCES

Bates, M. (1988) "State Zoning Legislation: A Purview." Wisconsin Council on Developmental Disabilities, Madison, Wisconsin.

Brody, E. (1981) "'Women in the Middle' and Family Help to Older People." Gerontologist, 21, 471-480.

Davis, K. (1983) "Financing Health Care for the Elderly in the U.S.: Current Policy Debate and Future Directions." Paper presented at the Commonwealth Fund Forum, London, England.

Federation Housing, Inc. (1988) "Conference on Aging in Place," Philadelphia, PA.

Granger-Jaffe, B. (1986) "Housing Report for Developers: A Survey of Housing Needs and Preferences of the Physically Disabled." Glenside, PA: Triad Assoc.

Hamlyn Associates (contracted by Pennsylvania Housing Finance Agency) (1989) "Supportive Services in Senior Housing Initiative." Research report published April 26, 1989 as part of a national study sponsored by the Robert Wood Johnson Foundation.

"A Health Profile of Older Pennsylvanians" (1988) Prepared by Pennsylvania Department of Aging and Pennsylvania Department of Health.

Longino, C. (1979) "Going Home: Aged Return Migration in the U.S., 1965-1970." *Journal of Gerontology, 34,* 736-745.

Lawton, M.P. (1986) *Environment and Aging.* (2nd Ed.) Center for the Study of Aging, Albany, New York (p. 137).

Lawton, M.P. & Hoover, S.L. (Eds.). (1981) Community Housing Choices for Older Americans. New York: Springer.

McGee and Associates (1988) "Market Study of Private Sector Senior Citizen Housing in the DuBois Pennsylvania Area." Dayton, OH.

Moore, J. (1986) "Building for Today's Retirement Markets: The Most Overlooked Market in the Industry" (Training Package) Moore Diversified Services, Inc., Fort Worth, Texas.

Newman, S. (1985) "The Shape of Things to Come." *Generations, 9* (3), 14-17.

Nwokeji, J., Schilling, D., Sanders-Jones, C. & Lamonto, S. (1988) "Service Assisted Housing," Pennsylvania Department of Aging.

"Pennsylvania's Growing Elderly Population" (1983) A brochure prepared by the Pennsylvania Department of Aging.

"A Profile of Older Americans: 1988" (1988) A pamphlet produced by American Association of Retired Persons and the U.S. Department of Health and Human Services/Administration on Aging, Washington, DC.

Pynoos, J. (1988) "Public Policy and Aging in Place: Identifying the problems and potential solutions" (Andrus Gerontological Center, University of Southern California). Paper presented at the National Conference on Support of the Frail Elderly in Residential Environments.

"Rental Retirement Housing: New Opportunities" (1986) Prepared for the National Corporation for Housing Partnerships (Washington, DC) by the Real Estate Research Corporation (Bethesda, MD).

"Service Assisted Housing Criteria" (1988) Pennsylvania Department of Aging.

Tiven, M. & Ryther, B. (1986) *State Initiatives in Elderly Housing: What's Tried and True.* Published by the Council of State Housing Agencies and National Association of State Units on Aging, Washington, DC.

"Understanding Senior Housing: An AARP Survey of Consumers' Preferences, Concerns, and Needs" (1989) American Association of Retired Persons, Washington, DC.

A Cost Comparison
of Congregate Housing and Long Term Care Facilities for Elderly Residents with Comparable Support Needs in 1985 and 1990

Leonard F. Heumann

The purpose of this paper is to determine if there are significant savings in housing frail but well elderly persons in long term care facilities or congregate living facilities. The paper updates to 1990 cost comparisons assembled from a sample of long term care and congregate facilities in 1985, and presented in a similar article describing the findings (Heumann, 1990).

Long term care facilities include nursing homes and homes for the aged, facilities designed to provide long term care for the chronically frail and ill who are incapable of independent living. Over the years, many of these facilities have adapted their policies to include elderly residents who are capable of assisted independent living. In part, this has been a response to the growing number of elderly without support and incapable of living in conventional housing. Depending on the local policy of long term care facilities and the availability of support services in the community, most studies estimate that between 20 and 25% of the elderly living

Leonard F. Heumann, PhD, is Professor of Urban and Regional Planning and the Housing Research and Development Program at the University of Illinois at Urbana-Champaign. He has conducted a wide variety of research in housing and community planning. For the last 16 years his research has focused on the housing needs of low-income and frail elderly persons with emphasis on improving market assessments of need, analyzing housing management alternatives, and cost comparisons between alternative housing options.

75

in long term care facilities could live in the community (Booz, Allan and Hamilton, 1975; Butler, 1975; Deetz, 1979; Kistin and Morris, 1972; Lawton, 1978; Thompson, 1979; Townsend, 1962; U. S. House, 1976). This is a significant percentage given the growing proportion of the population surviving to old age, especially if these elderly can live at a lower cost, with greater dignity and functional independence in the community.

Congregate housing provides the level of assisted, independent living that could meet the needs of elderly persons with chronic functional disabilities who are still capable of maintaining an independent apartment with support assistance. Congregate housing provides residents with independent apartments, at least one major meal served congregately per day, on-site social and laundry facilities, and the option of receiving assistance with additional meals, housekeeping, personal care, transportation and other support services if and when it is needed. No professional nurse or therapist is stationed on-site in a congregate facility. The typical on-site staff includes only a building manager, janitorial service and occasionally a social organizer. Congregate meals can be cooked on-site or catered. When support services are required, they are called in to provide support *at the margin of individual need*, rather than being provided institutionally. Elderly who require constant skilled surveillance or care would have to be transferred to a long term care facility. Studies of the elderly population indicate, however, that of the approximately 20% with chronic functional dependencies, more than two-thirds can live out their lives with the level of assisted independent living provided by congregate housing, while less than one-third require a long term, dependent living arrangement (Heumann and Boldy, 1982).

PREVIOUS COST COMPARISON RESEARCH

At one Congressional Hearing (U. S. House of representatives, 1981) congregate housing was reported to be approximately 40% less expensive to provide on a monthly basis than intermediate nursing home care. Another widely quoted study reported congregate housing could provide personal assistance and housekeeping for about $2-$5 per person per day in the mid 1970s, compared to $25-$30 in a local nursing home (Nachison, 1979).

Under Title IV of the 1978 Housing and Community Development Act, Congress authorized a federal Congregate Housing Services Program (CHSP), which provided subsidies of meals and support services to prevent frail elderly in subsidized housing from being transferred to nursing homes. This "demonstration program produced about 65 project sites nationwide" (Anderson, 1984). One study (Nenno et al., 1985, pp. 11-12) reported impressive monthly savings of $826 with the CHSP — over 300% cheaper than nursing home care.

There are currently 15 states with some form of congregate housing program, and four of the oldest (New Jersey, Connecticut, Maine and Massachusetts) have conducted cost comparison studies between their program and long term care with impressive savings accruing to the congregate housing facilities (Heumann, 1985; New Jersey, 1984; Gardner, 1984; Canale and Klinck, 1985; Commonwealth of Massachusetts, 1985; and Molica et al., 1984). There have been no comparative studies other than the one to be presented here since the mid-1980s, but new nationwide studies of elderly housing show that the provision of congregate services continues to grow in popularity (Gayda and Heumann, 1989; Gimmy and Boehn, 1988; and Struyk et al., 1989).

While almost all of the previous research uncovered shows cost savings with congregate housing, most of the studies *do not* control for comparable services to elderly with comparable support needs, nor do they always compare full housing and support service costs in both facilities. As a result, cost comparisons are not always accurate and often falsely exaggerate the savings in congregate living or the costs in long term care facilities.

THE MIDWEST COST COMPARISON STUDY

Cost comparison between congregate housing and long term care facilities presents a difficult and complex research problem. There are three basic reasons: first, the two types of facilities represent very different living environments (especially with regard to private accommodations); second, they represent very different support care alternatives (long term care uses on-site staff while congregate housing relies heavily on visiting services); and third, as indicated above, 75 to 80% of the long term care population on average are too frail to live in congregate housing, yet their support costs are often difficult to separate from the 20 to 25% who can transfer to congregate housing.

This study was designed to avoid the assumptions that limited the reliability and universality of the findings of previous studies. Undertaken first in 1985 and then repeated in 1990, the original study was designed to compare congregate housing and nursing homes in Illinois, but in 1985 there were too few congregate facilities in Illinois so a universe of seven midwest states was used: Illinois, Iowa, Michigan, Minnesota, Missouri, Ohio, and Wisconsin (Heumann, 1985).

The 1985 Research Design

The study was designed to look at all costs, subsidized and nonsubsidized, to the congregate housing and long term care facility residents that were not clearly identical for residents of both facility types. It also identified the universe of congregate and long term care facilities that were comparable by identifying facility characteristics that explained variations in cost of operation and services. Facilities selected for study were representative of the norm on these characteristics. Finally, the range of support service dependency in congregate housing was identified and costs derived by interviews with site managers. This was followed by interviews with long term care facility staff where costs were derived for residents with levels of support service dependency *comparable* to the congregate housing population.

Because of the depth of cost analysis and the need to choose both long term care and congregate housing sites with comparable residents, the sample universe had to be very carefully defined and stratified, and the study sites had to be limited to 14 (7 of each). In addition, it was necessary for facility owners to open their books and reveal detailed costs and charges. A high refusal rate was correctly anticipated, especially among for-profit facilities. Even after initial agreement and an in-depth site visit, one for-profit long term care facility sampled refused to release key cost figures and had to be dropped from the study reducing the long term care sites to six.

All facilities studied were limited to cities of 20,000 population or larger, located in counties defined as urban in the 1980 Census. This was necessary because of the significant differences in housing and support service character and cost, and support service availability between urban and rural areas, and the fact that the relatively small sample of sites being studied could not represent both urban and rural cost comparisons.

The 1990 Research Design

In 1990 a follow-up cost comparison was conducted by presenting the same 7 congregate facilities and 6 nursing homes with the cost figures generated in 1985, and asking each facility to update their expenses and income for all housing and support services. This was done by telephone and mail rather than site visits. The ranges of support dependency defined by the site managers in 1985 were retained in the 1990 follow-up to assure comparability of resident housing and support costs.

THE CONGREGATE HOUSING SAMPLE

In addition to the urban focus, eligible congregate facilities were limited to single buildings, with private apartments for residents (bedroom or studio style, private lavatory with bath or shower and private kitchen area), no entry fee or endowment, a minimum package of congregate services and spaces (one hot meal daily served in congregate dining and provision for other homemaker and personal care services as needed), and basic barrier-free and security design. This is by far the most common style of congregate housing in the Midwest and eliminates wide variation in the amount and type of living space the residents receive and are required to maintain.

A total of 55 congregate facilities fitting the above criteria were identified in 1985. These were then stratified by two characteristics: ownership and facility size. Twenty-six percent of the sites were private for-profit with an average facility size of 152 units; 60% were not-for-profit private or religious affiliated owners, with an average facility size of 127 units; and 14% were government owned (public housing), with an average size of 122 units. The facilities sampled were limited to a size range of 75 to 225 units to control for economies-of-scale in management and support service costs and sampled in proportion to the three ownership types. Due to lack of cooperation with private for-profit owners, only one such facility instead of two were sampled and an extra private not-for-profit owner was included. In the initial cost study of 1985, the congregate facilities were visited prior to any sampling of long term care facilities in order to first establish the range of functional disability that could be accommodated in congregate housing.

Comparison of 1985-1990 Basic Facility Demographics

In contrast to the nursing home sample, described below, the congregate facilities were very stable over the five year interval 1985-1990. All seven facilities had all available units rented and had waiting lists. Four of the facilities still had the same site manager in 1990 as 1985. The seven sites represented 1035 units, an average of 148 units per site in 1985 and 145 units in 1990. Six of the sites kept the same size, the single for-profit facility was in the process of remodeling down from 160 smaller apartments to 138 larger, more modern, and presumably, more marketable apartments. Expenses increased 16.2% on average over the five year period for these congregate housing facilities, while income increased

15.9% (the difference being made up in a slight loss in profits or replacement revenue).

Very few support services are defined and standardized when a person enters congregate housing. The concept is not to provide a standardized level of service, but to introduce support at the margin at which individual residents need assistance with their own efforts to maintain an independent household. As a result, numerous cost assumptions are necessary. Figure 1 summarizes the three levels of support service costs uncovered in the 1985 study. All seven managers reconfirmed these three support service levels in the 1990 study.

FIGURE 1. Levels of Support Services in Congregate Housing

Level I: Baseline Congregate Support
These elderly people are the most independent and require only barrier-free and secure building design and congregate meals.
  1. Basic shelter costs (rent plus utilities)
  2. Full congregate meals cost (90 meals/month)
  3. Basic sundry household budget
  4. Self-administered laundry (8 loads per month)
  5. Public transportation (32 one-way trips per month)

Level II: Intermediate Congregate Support
In addition to Level I services, these elderly people require some weekly assistance with housekeeping, and door-to-door transportation.
  1. Basic shelter costs
  2. Full congregate meals
  3. Basic sundry household budget
  4. Self-administered laundry
  5. Specialized transportation--door-to-door service (16 one-way
        trips/month)
  6. Heavy housekeeping (8 hours per month)

Level III: Advanced Congregate Support
In addition to Level I services, these elderly people require almost daily housekeeping assistance, some personal care, and one or more visits per week to monitor a health condition or provide minor medical assistance.

  1. Basic shelter costs
  2. Full congregate meals
  3. Advanced sundry household budget
  4. Housekeeper administered laundry
  5. Specialized transportation--lift van (8 one-way trips per month)
  6. Heavy and light housekeeping (16 hours per month)
  7. Personal care (8 hours per month)
  8. Nursing care (4 hours per month)
  9. Any social recreation or counseling charges

Food Service Costs

Each congregate facility required different amounts of group meals per month above the minimum of one per day for eligibility in the study (the average remained 47 out of 90 meals per month in both 1985 and 1990). How residents received the remaining meals was also extremely varied (personal shopping and cooking, restaurants, meals-on-wheels, additional meals purchased from the congregate housing kitchen, meals cooked by visiting housekeepers, eating with relatives, etc.). Because long term care facilities provide and require all residents to take all meals as part of the monthly charges, an equivalent full 90 meals per month had to be derived for the congregate housing facilities even though this typically *increased* the costs of congregate housing for most residents. Where all meals were provided 5 days per week, the per meal cost was added in for weekend days. Where a facility provided only the main meal, the second and third meal costs were estimated using meal costs at facilities that did provide these meals, weighted by the differences in the main meal costs.

No extra costs were charged for special dietary meals at any of the congregate facilities. All seven congregate facilities reported they could provide special dietary modifications at no cost when the modification required was an adaptation of the regular meal being served (e.g., salt free, weighed portions for diabetics, puréed meats and vegetables, etc.). Residents requiring long term special dietary modifications that cannot be similarly accommodated would be required to leave congregate housing. (Diverticulitis is a common example of a long term ailment mentioned by several congregate facilities that could not be accommodated in congregate housing.)

In 1985 one site used an off-site caterer exclusively and two other facilities used partial catering; by 1990 all seven facilities did some of the cooking on-site. The facility that changed from catered to on-site cooking actually cut costs from $199 for 90 meals in 1985 to $191 in 1990. Overall, the costs of a monthly congregate dining charge increased 28% over the five year period, from an average of $209 in 1985 to an average of $268 in 1990.

Sundry Living Expenses

Sundry living expenses is a cost totally overlooked in previous cost comparisons between long term care and congregate housing. These are costs subsumed under the operating budget of long term care facilities because they are under the control of the housekeeping staff and not the residents. The resident of a long term care facility is not responsible for shopping for housekeeping provisions or for the upkeep of whatever private space and furniture they possess.

In congregate housing, the resident maintains an independent apartment and must provide all the sundry equipment and supplies needed for daily living. A budget for such supplies was calculated utilizing a sample household supply inventory and local market prices. These costs remained the same for Levels I and II residents. The average cost for all seven facilities was $19 per apartment per month in 1985 and $23 per month in 1990. The study assumed an initial supply of dishes, cooking utensils, cleaning equipment (e.g., a vacuum cleaner), flat linen, and medicine cabinet supplies. The per month costs cover replacement and maintenance of these supplies. At Level III the average cost increased to $60 per apartment per month in 1985 and $72 in 1990. This is based on the assumption that more specialized disposable items are required such as bed and chair pads and adult disposable diapers. Disposable paper products for incontinent residents were provided as part of the overall charge in the long term care facilities in the study.

Transportation Costs

Transportation is another difficult cost to determine for congregate housing residents. The fact that they are still active in the larger community, and most are mobile, means that a great variety of both local and long distance trips are taken each month. Some housing managers feel that most trips are not vital to functional independence, are a matter of personal choice and life style, and should, therefore, be excluded from these cost calculations, along with a number of other nonessential items that are a matter of personal discretion. The majority of managers, however, felt that the ability to venture out and control one's own shopping, banking, socializing, etc., was an essential characteristic of assisted independent living. This was considered so important that three of seven facilities owned or leased a van or limousine for the private use of facility residents in 1985 and continued to do so in 1990.

Each level of congregate support requires a different type and amount of transportation. Level I residents, according to the managers, use conventional means of transportation and make the most trips. As summarized in Figure I, Levels II and III residents require more specialized transportation, but venture out less often, according to the managers. As a result, average monthly costs actually decline from $10 to $6 to $3 across the three support levels in 1985. These costs increased between 80% and

133% between 1985 and 1990 to $18 per month at level I, $14 at level II, and $7 at level III.

Housekeeping and Personal Care

The housekeeping and personal care services provided at congregate housing facilities are primarily from family, friends, and private agents hired by the resident or peripatetic community vendors. In 1985, a number of facilities provided on-site services or contracted with a single outside service vendor on behalf of all the tenants. This pattern has changed dramatically in five years, with most communities now implementing a "case management" program run through a social service agency or hospital, which screens people for eligibility and advises them on available services from a variety of vendors.

The cost of community service vendors is the logical common source of support to include in this study, however pricing their services requires another policy assumption. Most community services are nonprofit agencies subsidized by government grants and/or public contributions. Therefore, they not only charge on a sliding scale, but charges are subsidized for all recipients. The study could derive costs by using either the charge to the resident for a service or the real cost to provide the service. In all cases, *this study uses the average vendor charge to the resident* because these services represent a community commitment to assist tax paying residents of the community. They are often not services unique to the elderly, and certainly not unique to congregate housing. A visiting public nurse, homemaker or transportation service is available to any community resident who can benefit from the service. Since the elderly residents of the community have paid into the tax system and contributed to community fund raising over a lifetime, they have, and in effect are, paying their fair share of the actual provider cost.

For eight hours of service per month, average housekeeping costs rose 64% over the five years, from $22 to $36. In contrast, the average cost of eight hours of personal care declined 16% between 1985 and 1990. In part this was due to one facility, which participates in the federal Congregate Housing Services Program, changing to a flat fee charge to all residents for services in 1990, whether or not the residents used the services. This lowered individual costs of service users who were subsidized by non-user fees. Another reason for lower costs may have been that the new case management program and competing vendors produced cost efficiencies in 1990 that did not exist in 1985 (however some experts warn that this competition may have also lowered the quality of service).

Nursing, Counseling and Social Activity Costs

There were no user charges at any of the facilities for residents using visiting nurses services or personal counseling services in either 1985 or 1990. Social activity fees were charged by some park districts and when special site staff were hired. This amounted to $5 per month on average and did not change between 1985 and 1990.

Interpreting the Three Levels
of Support Dependency

Before discussing the long term care sample studied, it is important to understand what the three levels of support (summarized in Figure 1) represent for the cost analysis. Congregate housing sites in the Midwest, and indeed nationally, are relatively new and still have relatively young and independent populations. Most of the sites are still below the average resident age and average level of resident assistance at which they will stabilize in years to come. In the 1990 study, the average congregate housing facility studied reported that 80.7% of the residents were at level I, 14.5% were at level II, and 5% were at level III. As a result, the support profile of the average resident in the typical congregate facility today is likely to be Level I. To assume costs for congregate housing residents will remain at level I, however, is unrealistic and an unfair cost comparison with long term care facilities.

Despite their relative newness, this study also discovered that several congregate facilities already had one or two residents who were more dependent than the Level III definition of advanced congregate support. In the course of evaluating these congregate facilities, however, it became clear that the facilities could only accommodate the most severely frail and dependent elderly on a short term (3-6 months) or episodic basis, and then only a very small percentage of their total population could have such advanced and demanding dependencies. Therefore, it would be equally unrealistic to determine costs based on the most dependent elderly residing in congregate housing. Level III was established by identifying the most advanced level of support to which the *entire* population of congregate housing could evolve while still maintaining an assisted independent living environment for all residents without changing the on-site support staff in size or character. In conclusion, these three levels represent distinct changes in the level of care and support services provided to residents, as observed in the congregate housing site interviews, but none of the levels represent the true *norm* among congregate housing residents today. They were created to represent a fair cost range in cost comparisons with long term care facilities.

THE LONG TERM CARE SAMPLE

It was possible to focus entirely on Illinois long term care facilities since there were 1072 state-licensed facilities in 1985. The universe from which the study sample was drawn was narrowed down to 330 facilities in order to make fair and accurate comparisons with the congregate housing sample. Along with restriction to urban areas described above, five variables define long term care facilities as used in this study: type of licensing, type of ownership, building age, number of beds, and average facility cost per resident per day.

Facilities licensed for child care and developmentally disabled care were eliminated for the obvious reason that they do not focus predominantly on the elderly. Facilities licensed exclusively for skilled care were eliminated because residents at this stage of advanced medical dependency cannot live in congregate housing. On the advice of the Illinois Department of Public Health, facilities that were exclusively licensed for sheltered care residents were eliminated because Illinois facilities with this single licensure tend to house a disproportionate number of mentally disabled residents (elderly and nonelderly) with special care needs that are not duplicated in congregate housing. This left four combinations of licensed facilities containing subsets of residents with dependency characteristics similar to residents of congregate housing. These were facilities licensed to house: skilled, intermediate, and sheltered care; skilled and intermediate care; intermediate and sheltered care; and intermediate care only.

Ownership type was also considered, using the same breakdown as congregate housing: (1) for-profit, (2) not-for-profit, and (3) government facilities (e.g., county nursing homes). By cross-tabulating the three ownership types and the four licensure types, a 12 celled matrix showing the proportion of sites to be sampled was attained. Unfortunately, the two largest cells were for-profit skilled nursing and intermediate care facilities (44.5%) and for-profit intermediate care facilities (26.1%). There was such a high rate of refusal to cooperate among these for profit facilities that they had to be replaced with not-for-profit sites. Average number of beds reflects facility size and economies-of-scale and efficiency in staffing, administrative and operating costs. The weighted mean score for the universe was 157 beds and the range of weighted means among license and ownership types was quite broad (95 to 285). Sampled sites were kept within this range.

Age of the facility instead of average age of the residents was used because long term care facilities tend to be older and more established institutions and the average age of residents is very similar across facilities. More important to the study of capital costs (discussed below), is that the buildings studied be near the mean age for the sample universe, which was 22 years. Average age of the facilities studied was between 16 and 24 years.

Average cost per person per day is the most direct way to be sure that a sampled long term care facility is not skewed toward one cost extreme or the other. All facilities sampled were within $3.50 of the weighted mean daily cost according to data provided by the Illinois Department of Public Aid.

All the site visits to the long term care facilities sampled in 1985 began after the congregate housing site visits were completed and the three levels of congregate support were defined. It was already clear at that point that Level I residents were not included in most long term care facilities. Because of the institutionalized nature of both service provision and cost accounting in long term care facilities, it was *not* possible to separate costs at different levels of support similar to congregate housing. The respondents to the long term care facility questionnaire were able to identify the number of residents that fit in the Level II-III support range, and were able to provide a single set of costs for the type and amount of services in this range. This method of costing services was retained in 1990, except that all data was collected by mail instead of site visits.

Comparison of 1985-1990 Facility Demographics

The total beds (1142) and the average number of beds per facility (190) were the only demographics that remained the same between 1985 and 1990 for the nursing homes sampled. A general decline in financial viability of the sampled facilities seems to reflect unscientific reports about the entire industry. Three facilities showing profits or replacement revenues in 1985 underwent or are undergoing financial restructuring entering 1990. One not-for-profit facility was sold to a for-profit buyer who refused to reveal detailed cost/income figures for 1990. The other two had deficits of $799 and $420 per resident per month in 1990. The average facility had 20% vacant beds in 1985, this climbed to 33% in 1990. The average facility had 37% "case study residents" in 1985 (i.e., residents that were comparable in support services received by congregate housing residents); this declined to 28% in 1990. Finally, on average, 25% of the case study residents were public aid recipients in 1985; this declined to just 13% in 1990. Overall, expenses increased 49.9% in five years for the five long term care facilities reporting, compared to incomes which increased only 28.8% (the reader will recall that the congregate facilities sampled reported an average increase in expenses and incomes of about 16% between 1985 and 1990).

DAILY LIVING AND SUPPORT COSTS
EXCLUDED FROM THE STUDY

Certain costs were found to be identical for long term care and congregate housing residents in the 1985 field study, or could be assumed to be identical and therefore excluded from the cost comparison. These costs were:

1. Medical costs from a private physician, clinic or hospital. It was assumed that this is paid separately in both types of facility and usually covered by Medicare, Medicaid, or private insurance.
2. Cost for prescription medicines, for reasons similar to those discussed for physician costs.
3. Clothing. For the same level of functional independence and activity, clothing needs and costs in both congregate housing and long term care facilities should be the same.
4. Out of town travel and private entertainment. These costs are quite variable from person to person, and no meaningful average can be calculated.
5. Nonessential sundry items. Residents of both facility types can be expected to purchase candy, soft drinks, magazines, newspapers, etc., in equal amounts.
6. Hair care and podiatry. Similar costs for these services were collected at all sites in 1985.

COST COMPARISON
USING EXISTING DEBT SERVICES

Figure 2 shows the yearly savings with congregate housing using existing debt service to determine rent levels.

Income in long term care facilities is limited to one fee per resident per month. There are, however, two sources of income: private pay residents, where the rate and number of private pay residents is set by the facility,

FIGURE 2. Yearly Savings to Congregate Housing Using Existing Debt Service to Determine Rent Levels

	Charges Per Person Year		Savings Per Person Year[1]		Total Charges Per Facility Year[a] (in millions)		Savings Per Facility Year[1]	
	1985	1990	1985	1990	1985	1990	1985	1990
Private pay rate in long term care facilities	$11,136	$13,788			$1.65	$2.04		
Congregate Housing charges:								
Level I	$ 7,980	$ 9,852	$3,156	$3,936	$1.85	$1.46	$467,088	$582,582
Level II	$ 8,172	$10,176	$2,964	$3,612	$1.21	$1.51	$438,672	$534,576
Level III	$ 9,192	$11,400	$1,944	$2,388	$1.36	$1.69	$287,712	$353,424
Long term care facility charges with actual private pay/public aid mix	$ 9,942	$12,228			$1.41	$1.81		
Congregate Housing charges:								
Level I	$ 7,980	$ 9,852	$1,512	$2,376	$1.18	$1.46	$223,776	$351,648
Level II	$ 8,172	$10,176	$1,320	$2,052	$1.21	$1.51	$195,360	$303,696
Level III	$ 9,192	$11,400	$ 300	$ 828	$1.36	$1.69	$ 44,400	$122,544

1. Savings are derived by subtracting congregate housing charges from long term care charges.
2. Total facility charges are derived by multiplying per person charges for long term care and congregate facilities by the average number of units (148) in the congregate facilities sampled in 1985.

and public aid residents, where reimbursement rates are set by the state. The top half of Figure 2 uses the private pay rate. This is shown because the majority of case study residents (75% in 1985 and 86% in 1990) are private pay. A more accurate and fair income per case study resident, however, would be to add private pay, and the much lower public aid, case study residents at each facility and derive an average actual income per case study resident used in the bottom half of Figure 2. The public aid rate by itself is not included, because this rate does not support the case study residents. Depending on the type of care license in each long term care facility, public aid residents are subsidized by private pay and/or public aid residents receiving a higher level of care.

The congregate housing costs are defined to represent private pay insofar as construction and management cost of the facility are concerned. There are several subsidies not shown, such as low interest construction loans for some facilities and numerous community subsidies for visiting support services to individual residents. There are, however, similar subsidies to long term care facilities using the private pay rate. Most of these facilities are not-for-profit and receive property tax write-offs and favorable construction loans.

The reader is also reminded that the researchers sought costs from both types of facility at all three levels of support. This was not possible given the management and billing procedures in long term care facilities. As a result, Figure 2 compares a broad mean charge for all case study residents of the long term care facilities studied, with three different levels of congregate support costs, none of which is truly representative of the average costs in congregate housing.

Cost comparisons using Level I support costs artificially favors congregate housing because this is the least expensive support cost level, yet the typical congregate facility will not retain a majority of residents at such a high level of functional independence over the life of the facility.

Cost comparisons using Level III congregate housing service costs artificially favors the long term care facilities because, based on site observations, case study residents in long term care are not concentrated at Level III. If all their case study residents were to reach Level III status, the typical long term care facility would have much higher internal support costs and would most likely have to make financial adjustments by shifting some of the case study residents to a higher care level (and charge rate), and/or increasing the ratio of private pay residents. In fact, the latter has apparently happened in several facilities between 1985 and 1990.

The single best comparison would be the range of cost differences created by comparing Level II congregate housing charges with both private pay and private pay/public aid mixed charges for long term care. This comparison produces a savings per person per year of $1,320 to $2,964 for residence in congregate housing in 1985. This rises to a savings per person per year of $2,052 to $3,612 in 1990. On a total facility basis, the savings per year ranges from $195,360 to $438,672 with congregate housing in 1985, and $303,696 to $534,576 in 1990. This amounts to a 22% increase in savings over this five year period by placing private pay case study residents in congregate housing, and an increase in savings of 56% using the actual private pay/public aid mix of incomes for case study residents.

Two additional discussions are necessary to get a complete cost comparison. One is a refinement of the costs in Figure 2 normalizing capital costs and debt service. The second is reexamining the quality of life factors associated with living in congregate housing and long term care facilities which cannot be priced.

NORMALIZED CAPITAL COSTS AND DEBT SERVICE

The savings shown in Figure 2 are considered a very conservative estimate because the congregate facilities tended to be built after 1980 and the long term care facilities before 1970. This results in higher capital costs and debt service for congregate facilities. Normalizing capital costs and debt service to the present for all facilities results in a fairer comparison and simulates the cost of building new long term care or congregate living facilities in today's construction and service cost market.

Fundamental to normalizing costs is the replacement value for the reporting facilities based on the most recent insurance underwriting assessments of the value of the building and its contents. When this figure is standardized per bed in long term care facilities and per apartment in congregate housing, the per unit replacement value is almost identical among the sampled facilities—$41,691 per bed and $39,401 per apartment in 1985 and $52,356 per bed and $50,345 per apartment in 1990. The five year rates of inflation in these insurance underwriting assessments were almost identical—26% for long term care facilities and 28% for congregate housing facilities. The average congregate housing per unit replacement value of $50,345 in 1990 is quite reasonable and cost competitive with conventional apartment construction in the midwest. It is a particularly attractive price given that this replacement cost includes both a private apartment and a proportional share of congregate dining, social lounges, laundry room, and craft and recreation rooms. On the other hand, the $52,356 per bed figure for long term care includes no totally private space and relatively little communal space unique to the case study residents. The per bed replacement cost does include communal space that must be divided among various care classifications, as well as space exclusive to the extensive on-site support and administrative staff. In the facilities that house skilled care residents, this per bed replacement cost also represents more stringent and costly building construction standards, furniture, and equipment that is required by law in nursing care facilities.

In order to determine current capital costs and debt service, a multiplier was created based on prevailing mortgage interest rates and amortization periods for 1985 and 1990. The multiplier times the replacement value gave a total debt for replicating each facility in 1985 or 1990. It was then assumed that all facilities could last 40 years without major alterations or replacements to the building. Total debt service was divided by 40 years and by 12 months to get monthly debt service per unit assuming no vacancy rate. The existing debt service on each facility was then subtracted from any current debt service reported in facility expenses. The difference in monthly debt service per bed or apartment was treated as an added expense if these facilities were to be built and begin operation in 1985 or 1990. In order to maintain the profit margin or replacement revenue in each facility, this amount would also have to be added to the income side of the ledger and charged to each resident or apartment.

Figure 3 shows capital costs and debt service normalized to 1985 and 1990. With the same arguments used in describing Figure 2, the fairest comparisons are with Level II congregate housing charges, or a savings range of $4,233-$5,880 per resident per year if we were to build new congregate housing as opposed to long term care institutions in 1985. The savings increases to $4404-$5964 per resident per year if we were to build and begin operation of new congregate housing in 1990. Using the average 1985 facility size of the congregate housing surveyed (148 apartments), the savings from maintaining frail elderly persons in newly built congregate housing as opposed to newly built long term care institutions was $626,484-$870,240 per facility year in 1985 and $651,792-$882,672 in 1990.

While Figure 2 shows considerable savings in the operation of congregate housing over long term care for elderly persons of comparable support dependency, Figure 3 shows 65-115% greater savings with capital costs and debt service normalized to 1990 for both congregate and long term care facilities. The savings from new construction were even greater in 1985. This is because new mortgage interest rates on construction in May of 1985 were between 13.0% and 13.5% for most local housing

FIGURE 3. Savings to Congregate Housing with all Capital Costs and Debt Service Normalized to 1985 and 1990

	Charges Per Person Year		Savings Per Person Year[1]		Total Charges Per Facility Year[2] (in millions)		Savings Per Facility Year[1]	
	1985	1990	1985	1990	1985	1990	1985	1990
Private pay rate in long term care facilities	$16,788	$17,706			$2.49	$2.63		
Congregate Housing charges:								
Level I	$10,716	$11,460	$6,072	$6,300	$1.59	$1.70	$898,656	$932,400
Level II	$10,908	$11,796	$5,880	$5,964	$1.61	$1.75	$870,240	$882,672
Level III	$11,928	$13,020	$4,860	$4,740	$1.77	$1.93	$719,280	$701,520
Long term care facility charges with actual private pay/public aid mix	$15,141	$16,200			$2.24	$2.40		
Congregate Housing charges:								
Level I	$10,716	$11,460	$4,425	$4,740	$1.59	$1.70	$654,900	$701,520
Level II	$10,908	$11,796	$4,233	$4,404	$1.61	$1.75	$626,484	$651,792
Level III	$11,928	$13,020	$3,213	$3,180	$1.77	$1.93	$475,524	$470,640

1. Savings are derived by subtracting congregate housing charges from long term care charges.
2. Total facility charges are derived by multiplying per person charges for long term care and congregate facilities by the average number of units (148) in the congregate facilities sampled in 1985.

sponsors. The mortgage interest rates for the same sponsors dropped to between 10.5% and 11.25% in May of 1990. As a result, the savings shown in the previous paragraph that accrue to congregate housing from combining operating costs and normalized debt service increase only slightly between 1985 and 1990 (1.4% based on income from private pay residents of long term care and 4.0% on income from private pay/public aid mix).

TAKING A MORE CONSERVATIVE LOOK AT COST DIFFERENCES

A savings of $651,792 in just the first year of building one new congregate housing facility over building a new long term care facility of the same size to house elderly people of the same functional dependency level is a major savings. The fact that this savings has increased 4.0% for the actual mix of private pay and public aid resident despite the huge drop in mortgage interest rates between 1985 and 1990 is also remarkable. In the section to follow, this discussion of savings is expanded to consider all the non-quantifiable benefits that accrue with congregate living over institutionalization. Before proceeding, however, it might pay to take a more conservative look at the cost differences derived above. The most vulnerable element in this investigation is the small sample size. The detailed stratification of the sampling gave credibility to the initial sample chosen in 1985. The financial troubles faced by half the long term care facilities by 1990, however, may cause the reader to question the fairness of the follow-up cost comparison. This sample may not be representative of long term care facilities in 1990. Therefore, the cost comparison figures were reexamined using just the three long term care facilities that were able to keep up occupancy and hold the line on inflating costs.

When comparing the costs of the actual private pay/public aid mix for residents in these three long term care facilities with level II congregate housing residents, there was still a substantial savings of $577,200 per facility per year in 1990. This does, however, represent a decline of almost 8% in the savings from constructing new congregate housing in 1985 (when the savings was $626,484).

An interesting final note on these three most financially secure long term care facilities is that they represent the most heavily subsidized facilities, both in percentage of public aid and Medicaid certified case study residents, and construction and tax subsidies. Ironically, these are the very long term care facilities which may be denied the right to care for elderly persons in the range of support being discussed in this study due to 1987

OBRA (Omnibus Budget Reconciliation Act) legislation. While the regulations accompanying this legislation are still pending, preliminary OBRA regulations appear to require all long term care facilities that are Medicaid certified to discharge residents that do not require nursing care (Price, 1990). The logic behind this legislation is that long term care facilities are a cost ineffective place to house frail but well elderly — a finding this study supports.

QUALITY OF LIFE FACTORS

This concluding section repeats the conclusions presented in the 1985 study (Heumann, 1990), because the general quality of life and delivery of support in congregate housing and long term care institutions have not changed over the intervening five years.

One criticism of congregate housing is that it relies heavily on community provided visiting services that, if not present, are present only on weekdays, not of high quality, or not carefully monitored and coordinated, can result in *undercaring* of residents. While this criticism may be valid for some facilities, it was not a problem in the facilities sampled. This study was focused on urban areas with strong community peripatetic services. All the congregate facilities studied had staff trained to give counseling, information and referral, and had a monitoring system to check on residents daily.

Criticism of the quality of life in long term care facilities is far more extensive, especially when compared to the type of assisted independent living provided by congregate housing. Despite concerted efforts to identify and include the most progressive long term care facilities in this study sample, all long term care facilities limit the independence of residents when compared to congregate housing. At their worst, according to one study, they are custodial as opposed to rehabilitative environments that almost never provide or encourage independent living (Auston and Kasberg, 1976). They often can encourage "learned helplessness" and docile dependence on support staff (Mercer and Kane, 1979). This can result in rapid atrophy of physical and social skills, making long term care facilities a poor substitute for residents of similar support needs living in congregate housing.

The major differences were in the physical settings that comparable case study residents received in congregate housing and long term care. When comparing dining, the number of entree choices and choice of proportion sizes was very similar in both types of facility, as was the quality of food and menu ranges. The fact that all long term care facilities separate skilled, intermediate and sheltered care residents in different areas of the facility means that case study residents dine with others at their level of functional independence. Nevertheless, the congregate facilities tend to have dining rooms with less institutional appearance and provide more social flexibility and a more casual atmosphere for dining. More guests were seen attending meals in the congregate facilities, and more congregate housing residents at all levels of support were away from the facility at mealtime.

The bottom line in physical cost comparisons is that despite the considerably higher costs, the case study resident is getting much less in long term care. He or she receives 100-150 square feet of semiprivate space around a bed in a nursing institution compared to 400-500 square feet of private apartment in congregate housing.

Unlike most long term care facility residents, congregate housing residents retain control of their money, their personal affairs, their daily routine and the freedom to come and go as they please. Congregate housing appears to promote more self-sufficiency, encourage cost-saving interdependence with friends and neighbors in the facility and the community, offset social isolation and introduces costly professional support services only at the margin of individual needs.

The major reasons for the substantial costs savings with congregate housing are: (1) the elimination of expensive on-site nursing care, physical and occupational therapy, and personal care, and (2) the elimination of dependent living arrangements which do not promote self-sufficiency. Conversely, congregate housing is cost effective because it: (1) promotes independent living, (2) promotes self-sufficiency at the margin of individual ability to care for oneself and/or promotes interdependent support with friends and relatives in the private community (primarily other congregate housing neighbors), (3) promotes social engagement and activity, and (4) brings in professional support only at the margin of individual need. The key to low cost congregate living for most elderly persons is the successful combination of a supportive physical environment, personal capabilities employed to their fullest, and low skill on-site support services. For others, it is just the small amount of regular visiting professional services and personal care in addition to the on-site services that is the key to maintaining their independence.

This researcher strongly recommends that elderly persons with support needs that can be accommodated in congregate housing be provided congregate housing. This in no way implies that long term care facilities do not provide excellent and important care for elderly with advanced frailties who *require* a dependent support environment. To the best of their abilities, all the long term care facilities studied provided as pleasant an atmosphere as possible with caring and supportive staff. The fact remains, however, that it is almost impossible to provide both dependent and independent support environments under the same roof and by the same staff. The physical atmospheres and staff functions are in conflict. Despite best intentions, nursing institutions cannot serve as private homes. The level of state reimbursements to sheltered care residents as opposed to intermediate and skilled care residents is also in conflict. Sheltered care residents are reimbursed so much less, proportional to their support needs, that they become financially dependent on higher levels of care. This encourages either premature reclassification of sheltered care residents to higher care levels or lowering of sheltered care support quality.

REFERENCES

Anderson, E. "Report on the Congregate Housing Services Program," Public Housing Agency of the City of St. Paul, Minnesota, Unpublished Letter Report, April 1984.

Auston, M. and Kasberg, J. "Nursing Home Decision-Makers and the Social Service Needs of Residents." *Social Work in Health Care*, Vol. 1, 1976, pp. 447-56.

Booz, Allan, and Hamilton. *Long Term Care Study*. Volume II, State Department on Aging, Springfield, Illinois, 1975.

Butler, R. N. *Why Survive? Being Old in America*, Harper and Row Publishers, New York, 1975.

Canale, J. and Klinck, M. E. *Report of the Congregate Housing Study Committee*, Connecticut Department of Housing and Department on Aging, Hartford, April 1985.

Commonwealth of Massachusetts, *The 1984 Annual Report of the Executive Office of Elder Affairs*, The Commonwealth of Massachusetts, Boston, 1985.

Deetz, V. L. "Congregate Housing: A Growing Need." *HUD Challenge*, United States Department of Housing and Urban Development, Washington, DC, August 1979.

Gardner, A. *A Report on Maine's Congregate Housing Program*, Bureau on Maine's Elderly, Department of Human Services, Augusta, Maine, August 1984.

Gayda, K. S. and L. F. Heumann. *The 1988 National Survey of Section 202 Housing for the Elderly and Handicapped*, Subcommittee on Housing and Consumer Affairs, U.S. Congress, Washington, DC, December 1989.

Gimmy, A. E. and M. A. Boehn. *Elderly Housing: A Guide to Appraisal, Market Analysis, Development and Finance*, American Institute of Real Estate Appraisals, Chicago, 1988.

Heumann, L. F. *A Cost Comparison of Congregate Housing and Long Term Care Facilities in the Midwest*, Illinois Housing Development Authority, Chicago, Illinois. September 1985.

Heumann, L. F. "The Housing and Support Costs of Elderly with Comparable Support Needs Living in Long-Term Care and Congregate Housing." *Journal of Housing for the Elderly*, Vol. 6, Nos. 1 and 2, 1990, pp. 45-71.

Heumann, L. F. and Boldy, D. *Housing for the Elderly: Planning and Policy Formulation in Western Europe and North America*. St. Martins Press, New York, 1982, pp. 16-58.

Kistin, H. and Morris, R. "Alternatives to Institutional Care for the Elderly and Disabled." *Gerontologist*, Part I, Vol. 12, 1972, pp. 139-142.

Lawton, M. P. "Institution and Alternatives for Older People." *Health and Social Work*, Vol. 3, 1978, pp. 108-134.

Mercer, S. O. and Kane, R. A., 1979. "Helplessness and Hopelessness in the Institutionalized Aged: A Field Experiment." *Health and Social Work*, Vol. 4, pp. 90-116.

Molica, R. et al. *Congregate Housing for Older People: An Effective Alternative*. Final report. Massachusetts Department of Elder Affairs and Building Diagnostic, Inc., Boston, MA, June 1984.

Nachison, J. S. "Services for Congregate Housing: A New Direction for HUD." *HUD Challenge*, U. S. Department of Housing and Urban Development, Washington, DC, August 1979.

Nenno, M. K., Nachison, J. S., and Anderson, B. "Support Services for the Frail Elderly or Handicapped Persons Living in Government-Assisted Housing: A Public Policy Whose Time Has Come," working paper, February 1985.

New Jersey, Division on Aging, *Rules and Regulations: Congregate Housing Services Program*, Division on Aging, Congregate Housing Services Programs, April 1984.

Price, R. *Medicare and Medicaid Nursing Home Reform Provisions in the Omnibus Budget Reconciliation Act of 1987, P.L. 100-203*. Congressional Research Service Report for Congress 90-80EPW, Library of Congress, Washington, DC, August 10, 1989, Revised January 16, 1990.

Struyk, R.J. et al. *Providing Supportive Services to the Frail Elderly in Federally Assisted Housing*, Urban Institute Report 89-2, Washington, DC, June, 1989.

Thompson, M. M. "The Elderly in our Environment: Yesterday and Today." *HUD Challenge*, United States Department of Housing and Urban Development, Washington, DC, August 1979.

Townsend, P. *The Last Refuge*, Routledge and Kegan Paul, London 1962.

United States House of Representatives, Select Committee on Aging, Subcommittee on Housing and Consumer Interests. *Congregate Housing Services*, U.S.G.P.O., Washington, DC, 1981, p. 47.

United States House of Representatives, Select Committee on Aging, Subcommittee on Housing and Long Term Care. *New Perspectives on Health Care for Older Americans*. U.S.G.P.O., Washington, DC, January 1976.

Realities
of Political Decision-Making
on Congregate Housing

Donald L. Redfoot
Katrinka Smith Sloan

INTRODUCTION

One of the most enduring contributions of the phenomenological school of social science is the dislodging of the notion of a single "reality" that is taken for granted in everyday life. As Alfred Schutz noted, life experiences are divided into "multiple realities," each with its own "cognitive structure" (Schutz, 1973, pp. 207-59). Though any society represents a shared social reality without which social interaction would be impossible, experiences of that "reality" are highly varied depending on one's position within a social structure. In other words, different aspects of any social reality are more or less "relevant" depending on one's social position (see also Berger and Luckmann, 1966).

Donald Redfoot, PhD, is a legislative representative on housing and transportation issues with the American Association of Retired Persons (AARP). Previously, he served as a staff member to the House Aging Committee's Subcommittee on Housing and Consumer Interests, where he wrote a committee report on the Congregate Housing Services Program. In his pre-Washington career, Dr. Redfoot spent three years as a post-doctoral Fellow at the Aging Center at Duke University on grants form the National Institute for Mental Health and the National Institute on Aging. He also taught sociology courses with the European Division of the University of Maryland. Katrinka Smith Sloan, MA, is Assistant Manager of the Consumer Affairs Department of the American Association of Retired Persons. Previously, she worked as a Policy Research Specialist with the American Association of Homes for the Aging and as a Staff Assistant to Senator Thomas Eagleton. Ms. Sloan is the co-author (along with Ann Gillespie) of a recent book entitled *Housing Options and Services for Older Adults* (1990, ABC-Clio Press).

99

Legislative advocacy to address the needs of frail older people places one in a mediating position between the "reality" experienced by those older people and the very different "reality" experienced by political decision makers. Each reality has a completely different structure of relevance that becomes particularly apparent in the attempt to communicate and advocate on behalf of programs serving the frail. This article will describe this clash of relevance structures by focusing on the debate over one of the federal government's tiniest programs, the Congregate Housing Services Program (CHSP).

The Congregate Housing Services Program (CHSP) was established by Title IV of the Housing and Community Development Act of 1978 to provide nomedical services to residents of Section 202 and public housing for the elderly and handicapped. The mission of the CHSP was to "prevent the premature institutionalization" of residents. Due to budget constraints, the program was immediately scaled back to demonstration status. Currently, only sixty sites nationwide serve approximately 1800 frail older and disabled people.

In contrast to other articles in this volume, which concentrate on the "reality" experienced by the frail older person, this article will focus primarily on the "reality" experienced by political decision makers. Implications will be drawn in the conclusion for empowering older people. The authors' perspective for observing this clash of relevance structures has been as advocates on behalf of expanding congregate services. While this perspective gives access to both worlds, the advocacy role admittedly colors the view of the policy debates described below.

Three themes will resurface throughout the discussion of the relevance structure through which decision makers view congregate services. First, the overwhelming reality in any Congressional discussion is the budget constraint imposed by a combination of the massive deficits of the 1980s and the resulting Gramm-Rudman-Hollings deficit targets. No matter what the merits of any program, the first (and often the last) question asked is, "What does it cost?"

Second, the discussions around congregate services are still largely framed by the institution-based, long-term care system which has had a distorting effect on discussions of the effectiveness and cost of congregate services. This point is largely corollary to the first since the current and projected costs of Medicaid-funded long-term care have been driving the search for alternatives, among which is congregate housing.

Third, scholars who venture into "policy relevant" work should be forewarned that their work will be shamelessly used and misused as ammunition in political battles. The debates among decision makers in Congress and the Administration are over allocation of scarce resources they are not exercises in seeking truth.

HOUSING-BASED VS. INSTITUTION-BASED: THE JURISDICTIONAL BATTLES

One of the most important elements of the relevance structure of decision makers is jurisdiction. Early proponents of congregate housing attempted to break through the institutional lock on definitions of long-term care by emphasizing *housing* as the core service of congregate living, thereby defining its legislative and programmatic jurisdiction. Albert Eisenberg, who as a Congressional staff member helped draft the enacting legislation, explained at a 1985 hearing:

> We decided to give the program to HUD. We viewed it as a housing program, not a services program. Unfortunately, all the people who seem to review this in the administration circles are all on the services side rather than on the HUD side. When it got up to OMB, at the time we put forth this program, it went to the services people who did not understand it. It is a housing program. It gives people a type of living situation that they could not otherwise have. (U.S. Select Committee on Aging, 1985, p. 59)

The emphasis on housing was to reinforce the intention of the program to maximize independent living. As Eisenberg put it more succinctly in a recent conversation, "If you give the program to HHS, they'll have the participants in bathrobes and wheelchairs in no time." As anecdotal support of his position, we recently reviewed a proposed piece of legislation which came to us from the committee staff of a leading U.S. Senator. As part of a bill to integrate housing and services, provisions were incorporated that would give jurisdiction for services to the frail and disabled to an office within the Department of Health and Human Services. The first eligible service listed was "24-hour nursing supervision services," a move that could trigger nursing home regulations and transform housing projects into nursing homes almost overnight.

With impeccable logic and reams of research, scholars could debate the merits of housing-based versus institution-based services to the frail and disabled. Simply noted here, however, is that all of that research and logic may have little to do with the outcome of the political battle because of powerful jurisdictional and institutional barriers to a housing-based policy for serving people with disabilities. These barriers come from both the housing and services sides, reflecting entrenched definitions of long-term care responsibilities.

As the recent scandals have all-too-clearly revealed, HUD is an institution governed by a "bricks and mortar" mentality — where financing and development issues take precedence over broader policy concerns for the housing and community needs of human beings. The bricks and mortar mentality extends not only to those whose greed has recently been exposed. Even those concerned for the plight of the poor and ill-housed have been quick to argue that the provision of services is not HUD's business. As one spokesman explained HUD's opposition to expansion of congregate services, "The fact is, however, that the housing programs under HUD are just that — housing. The housing built under Section 202 was never oriented to care (U.S. House Committee on Aging, 1988)."

This attitude is not entirely partisan, nor confined to the Administration. Congressional discussions are also driven by concerns other than a burning desire to know the best possible way to overcome jurisdictional barriers in order to serve those needing assistance. The CHSP is no exception to the general questions, "What does it cost?" and "Who pays?" More will be said about the first question below. For now, a few observations will be made about "who pays?" as a major concern behind the jurisdictional battles.

Much of the motivation for establishing the CHSP in the first place was the belief that federal Medicaid dollars could be saved by preventing unnecessary institutionalization in nursing homes. However, even if we assume for the moment that significant savings would accrue from a policy shift from institution-based to housing-based services, opposition would still result because the costs are borne by one agency or level of government while the savings accrue in another agency or level of government. One influential Congressional staff person has said that he could not help obtain more CHSP funding because the money would come out of the HUD budget while the savings would accrue to Medicaid.

A similar argument holds with regard to the division of responsibility among levels of government. For example, subsidies for services in congregate or "sheltered" housing in many areas come entirely from state and local budgets, while nursing home costs for the poor are split by federal and state governments under Medicaid. Because state and local governments receive no reimbursement for congregate services, Heumann et al., (1985, p. 62) report that sheltered housing residents are "prematurely transferred to intermediate care in order . . . to receive a realistic reimbursement rate."

On the other hand, a proposal to share the cost of an expanded CHSP with state and local governments could face complaints by the nation's governors that too much of the cost of federal programs and mandates is being passed on to the states. In short, even if both federal and state governments would gain from decreased Medicaid costs, larger jurisdictional battles could stymie efforts to expand congregate housing services.

It would be remiss if this section ended without noting a significant change in the attitude at HUD on the issue of its role in the provision of services. A newly expansive approach to housing and services is reflected in recently released housing reform proposals from HUD which would create major new services programs to assist the homeless with mental health and addiction services and young families in public housing with child care and job training. Unfortunately, apart from a tiny demonstration to link services with rental vouchers, HUD's proposals would do nothing to help frail older or disabled people. The President's budget for fiscal year 1991 proposes once again to eliminate the CHSP, as has every budget since fiscal year 1982.

DOES THE PROGRAM WORK?
A LESSON IN THE POLITICS
OF DATA MANIPULATION

The charge to "prevent premature institutionalization" has defined the CHSP, even if negatively, in terms of an institutional model of long-term care. Those who wrote the legislation could have framed the discussion in terms of promoting independence or preventing more likely alternatives such as living with relatives or suffering in isolation. Even outcomes of interest to decision makers such as preventing or shortening acute care were ignored.

Whether or not the CHSP has been successful in preventing premature institutionalization would seem to be a relatively straightforward question. However, in addition to the usual scholarly qualifications which make straight answers to policy questions rare, assessment of congregate services has suffered more than usual from partisan manipulation of "independent" research.

In an unusual moment of sound research policy on program effectiveness, Congress required that an independent evaluation of the CHSP be conducted when the program was enacted. To meet this mandate, HUD contracted with the Hebrew Rehabilitation Center for the Aged in Boston to conduct a study that was initiated in 1980 and completed in 1985 (Sherwood et al., 1986).

Samples were drawn from 17 CHSP awardee sites and from carefully matched facilities without CHSP services. Information was gathered at three points in time. The first or "Baseline" round of questioning was conducted before the program began to offer services. Reflecting a lag between baseline and actual program initiation, the second round of questioning—described in the report as " Wave I"—was conducted an average of 14 months after baseline, but actually covered only 8 to 10 months of program experience. Finally, a more cryptic third round of interviews, or "Wave II," was conducted by telephone approximately one year later.

The researchers found that between Baseline and Wave I, 7% of the CHSP "Experimentals" and 9% of the non-CHSP "Controls" had spent time in institutional care, a statistically insignificant difference. However, during the period between Waves I and II, 18% of the "Controls" versus only 10% of the "Experimentals" had been institutionalized, a difference that is significant both to statisticians and to decision makers. In addition, the report noted that managers of CHSP sites were six times more likely to accept new residents from nursing homes than those managers who had no such services to offer, indicating a strong deinstitutionalization effect (Sherwood et al., 1986).

These data would seem to indicate a highly successful program. Nonetheless, in conveying the final report to Congress in 1986 (one year after its completion), Secretary Samuel Pierce reported the astonishing conclusion, "In summary, the results show that CHSP worked well administratively, but was not successful in achieving its primary goal of preventing premature institutionalization" (U.S. House Select Committee on Aging, 1988, p. 149).

To understand this conclusion requires knowledge of the events that occurred in the year between the submission of the final report to HUD by the independent researchers and its release to Congress. In order to control information disseminated by the Administration, all such reports are reviewed by the Office of Management and Budget (OMB) prior to their release. After an initial review before sending the report to OMB, HUD had recommended only minor editorial changes in what was—apart from criticisms of the program's targeting—a very positive report. OMB returned the report to HUD with a letter (leaked to Congressional staff) suggesting major "edits" in the final report to make it conform to Administration policy. As the letter stated (U.S. House Select Committee on Aging, 1988, p. 91):

In general my edits are an effort to give the report a more objective tone. For example, I would change terms like "highly successful" throughout where this is not borne out by hard data or is subject to subjective judgement. . . .

Secondly, I feel strongly that the report should not make statements that are contrary to policy. For example, the paragraph that talks about how the program will get better targeted as the result of regulatory change seems irrelevant if HUD is proposing to discontinue the program. . . .

Finally, I want to ask whether or not the Executive Summary or the transmittal letter should not make the case for the Administration's decision to discontinue Congregate Services more explicitly.

True to orders, HUD rewrote the final report and executive summary to reflect the Administration's policy, changes thoroughly documented in a House Aging Committee report. Parallel passages from the two versions of the executive summary summarize the changing verdict on the program's effectiveness (U.S. House Select Committee on Aging, 1988, p. 251):

The Original Draft

The Year Two findings suggest that this program can have positive effects on institutionalization. However, this potential is masked to some extent by the relatively small group of people who were likely to be institutionalized at Baseline. Such a result might be more easily accomplished if, for example, public housing projects set aside certain buildings for the most needy and vulnerable. Private sponsors as well should be encouraged to develop housing focused primarily on the more at-risk population. . . . Such targeting would strengthen and help CHSP-type programs to achieve their goals in an efficient manner.

OMB Approved Version

In conclusion, while CHSP was relatively successful in some measures (e.g., targeting, ease of implementation) it was not successful in achieving its primary goal—preventing premature institutionalization.

Note that neither HUD nor the independent researchers dispute that, on the whole, those receiving the services really needed them. Nor did either dispute the fact that the lives of those receiving the services were enriched and their independence enhanced. Moreover, HUD did not dispute the finding that CHSP services seem to provide an important respite to families. Since the program's success or failure was defined in terms of its ability to prevent institutionalization, HUD selectively reported the results and proclaimed the program a failure.

HUD's conclusion about the failure of the program, though discredited, has had a continuing negative effect on the program. The House Aging Committee's Subcommittee on Housing and Consumer Interests launched an investigation that documented the changes in the CHSP report and held a hearing at which scholars and practitioners, including a principal investigator from the Hebrew Rehabilitation Center, attested to the effectiveness of the program. Nonetheless, HUD's fiscal year 1991 budget recommends no funding because "the demonstration had little impact on preventing the institutionalization of these individuals" (U.S. Department of Housing and Urban Development, 1990, p. H-59).

IS THE CHSP COST EFFECTIVE?

The pernicious effect of using institution-based long-term care approaches to define the "relevant" dimensions of the policy debate over congregate services is nowhere more apparent than in discussions of the "cost effectiveness" of the CHSP. Normally, cost effectiveness would be measured by establishing a clear goal and comparing the cost of different approaches to fully accomplishing the goal.

By this definition, the cost effectiveness of the CHSP relative to nursing home care would be measured by comparing the cost of adequately serving similarly disabled people in different settings. The most persuasive scholarly study structured to compare congregate versus nursing home services in this way was conducted at the University of Illinois under the direction of Professor Leonard Heumann. Controlling for factors such as level of disability and relative capital costs, their study concluded that congregate services could be offered at a savings of 28-35% ($4,233-$5,880 per person per year in 1985 dollars) when compared to nursing home care.

While these conclusions are part of the public record, they are also considered largely beside the point by many decision makers. Everyone, including HUD and OMB, will agree that a hypothetical frail individual could receive congregate services at a cost that is less than nursing home care. What is relevant to decision-makers, however, is how to save Medicaid dollars likely to be spent on nursing home care in the face of large projected increases. This question requires moving the level of analysis from an individual to an aggregate comparison of the costs of alternative service delivery mechanisms.

At the aggregate level, the issue of saving federal Medicaid dollars is highly sensitive to the targeting of the services. Since we know who is served by Medicaid, saving money requires that congregate services be targeted to just those who would otherwise require Medicaid-funded nursing home care. There are no data which would definitively answer the question of whether such savings are possible. Several requests by the Hebrew Rehabilitation Center to extend their research to this question were denied by HUD.

To illustrate the sensitivity of the cost argument to targeting, however, these researchers put together some "back-of-the-envelope" numbers illustrating the poor potential for savings if few project residents are at risk of institutionalization (U.S. House Select Committee on Aging, 1988, p. 78). Like the conclusions on the program's effectiveness, the cost section of their final report was distorted beyond recognition by the HUD editors. As finally released, this illustration was transformed into a cost comparison between congregate services and nursing home care. The numerous errors of logic, data, and mathematics that further distort the analysis are detailed in the Aging Committee report (U.S. House Select Committee on Aging, 1988, pp. 215-21).

Of relevance to decision makers was the conclusion manufactured at HUD: "CHSP, as a program, proved to be more expensive than nursing home care" (Ibid., p. 250). A draft annual report on the CHSP that was leaked to Congress a year later made the further claim that, "The CHSP was three times as costly for the Federal Government than to simply institutionalize those residents of HUD projects when they need nursing home care" (Ibid., p. 252). While this conclusion is hopelessly inaccurate, it is nonetheless now entrenched as OMB dogma.

As advocates of the program, it would be desirable to report that definitive proof exists that money can be saved by more extensive use of congregate services. A more usable framing of the argument for decision makers, however, was offered by Newman and Struyk (1987), who calculated approximately how narrowly targeted a program of congregate services would have to be in order to break even with the expected rate of institutionalization. They suggest that 145 to 195 persons could be served in congregate housing for the same cost of serving 100 people in nursing homes.

Unfortunately, this targeting standard may be tough to meet. Even ignoring those who manage to get services but do not need them, there are two reasons why congregate services will serve a broader group than nursing homes. First, people will do most anything to avoid placement in a nursing home. In accounting terms, the savings from not serving those who have the same level of need but receive no government-reimbursed care accrue to the federal and state governments while the costs of our current system appear in the form of overtaxed families and friends and miserable lives for those unserved.

Second, congregate services should be targeted to those having less functional disability than those who would otherwise be in an institution, especially as the targeting of nursing home care is increasingly tightened. Congregate housing services should fill the gap in the continuum of care between fully independent living and nursing home care. Accordingly, the CHSP should be structured to allow early interventions designed to break the downward spiral that can lead to the nursing home.

In terms of the overall cost to the federal government, therefore, net savings are highly unlikely. Researchers could fill a major gap in our knowledge by documenting the marginal cost of filling in the continuum of care over the current system which largely reimburses only nursing home care. Such research should take into account the additional number of people who would be served, the consequences of such interventions on the lives of those served, and the delay in tapping the reimbursement stream under Medicaid and other programs. Decision makers would then have available the most honest data to frame discussions of future long-term care policy.

CONCLUSION

While one can be sympathetic to the budget problems facing Congress, casting the issue of congregate services in terms of Medicaid savings could have serious negative effects on policy discussions of long-term care alternatives. In this respect, the authors find themselves somewhat at odds with the researchers at the Hebrew Rehabilitation Center. The implication of their argument is that, in order to save money, congregate housing services should only intervene at an advanced state of disability, with more intensive services, in settings that concentrate on the frail and disabled. The effects of such a policy may make housing projects look increasingly like nursing homes.

One is reminded of the Vietnam commander who declared that he had to "destroy the village in order to save it." Some defenders of the program have argued, in essence, that the only way to save independent living for frail older people is to destroy the independent-living nature of the housing project. Such reasoning has already led HUD to narrow the targeting of the program from one problem with activities of daily living (ADL) to three — a very advanced state of disability that may mean interventions that are too late to be effective in preventing institutionalization. Congressional decision makers are afraid of loosening the targeting lest they undermine the cost saving argument. Sadly, by confining the discussion to terms established by institutional alternatives, the negative aspects of nursing homes may be replicated in congregate housing settings.

To come back to the original theme of multiple realities, note that the jurisdictional and budget constraints that define "reality" for decision makers have little to do with the "reality" experienced by frail older people in their daily lives. No departments of housing or human services divide the reality experienced by the older person whose independence is threatened by an inability to accomplish the tasks of everyday living. Budget deficits have no reality to the individual who is struggling to avoid costly and potentially confining nursing home care.

Similarly, the "realities" experienced by managers and providers differ from those experienced by either political decision makers or frail residents. Managers and providers play a mediating role between the reality experienced by the people they serve and the bureaucracies from whom they must receive their support. Very often this mediating role forces conflicting obligations between the roles as advocate for the service recipients and gatekeeper for the funding bureaucracy.

In order to be effective in overcoming jurisdictional and budgetary blinders, political advocacy for congregate services must refocus the policy discussions on the experiences of those who are served. Presentations of the life experiences of those whose lives have been affected by congregate services can be the most effective means to persuading those whose skepticism is based on jurisdictional or budgetary grounds. Until the reality experienced by the older person is considered paramount, progress will be difficult in expanding the federal commitment to congregate housing services.

RESOURCES

Berger, P. & Luckman, T. (1966) The Social Construction of Reality. New York: Doubleday.

Heumann, L., Rose, J., and Patton, T. (1985). *A Cost Comparison of Congregate Housing and Long-Term Care Facilities in the Midwest.* Report to the Illinois Housing Authority, Department of Research and Policy Development.

Newman, S. and Struyk, R. (1987). *Housing and Supportive Services: Federal*

Policy for the Frail Elderly and Chronically Mentally Ill. Washington, DC: Urban Institute.

Schutz, A (1973) Collected Papers. Vol. 1. The Hague, Netherlands: Martinus Nijhoff.

Sherwood, S., Morris, J., Sherwood, C., Morris, S., Bernstein, E., and Gornstein, E. (1986). *Final Report of the Evaluation of the Congregate Housing Services Program.* Prepared for the U.S. Department of Housing and Urban Development.

Struyk, R., Page, D., Newman, S., Carroll, M., Ueno, M., Cohen, B., and Wright, P. (1989). *Providing Supportive Services to the Frail Elderly in Federally Assisted Housing.* Washington, DC: Urban Institute.

U.S. Department of Housing and Urban Development (1990). FY 1991 Budget.

U.S. House Select Committee on Aging, Subcommittee on Housing and Consumer Interests (1985). Maximizing Supportive Services for the Elderly in Assisted Housing: Experiences from the Congregate Housing Services Program. Hearing Print.

U.S. House Select Committee on Aging, Subcommittee on Housing and Consumer Interests (1988). Dignity, Independence, and Cost Effectiveness: The Success of the Congregate Housing Services Program. Hearing Print.

III. PROGRAMMATIC PERSPECTIVES

Social Relations in Enriched Housing for the Aged: A Case Study

Lenard W. Kaye
Abraham Monk

Research findings to date tend to confirm positive effects of planned housing for the elderly on a variety of effectiveness measures, such as housing satisfaction, general life satisfaction, involvement in community and on-site activities, and the quality of socio-behavioral relations (Law-

Lenard W. Kaye, DSW, is Professor and Associate Dean at the Bryn Mawr College Graduate School of Social Work and Social Research in Bryn Mawr, PA. Abraham Monk, PhD, is Professor of Social Work at the Columbia University School of Social Work in New York City.

A modified version of this paper was presented at the 40th Annual Scientific Meeting of the Gerontological Society of America, Washington, DC, November 20, 1987. Support for this study was provided by the Brookdale Endowment of UJA-Federation of Jewish Philanthropies of New York and Jewish Association for Services for the Aged (JASA), New York, NY.

The authors express appreciation to Dr. Beverly Diamond, Research Associate, who played an important role in the collection and analysis of the original data for this study.

111

ton and Cohen, 1974; Carp, 1976; Sherwood, Greer and Morris, 1979; Lawton, 1982; Hinrichsen, 1985; Sherman, 1985; Select Committee on Aging, 1988). Furthermore, many older heads of households express strong interests in one or more of the non-traditional planned housing alternatives. Turner and Magnum (1982) report that one-third of home-owners interviewed in a national study of 1304 older householders residing in non-institutional arrangements were interested in housing which offers personal care services, and 6 to 8 percent were interested in such options as reverse annuity financing, partial conversion of the home into rental units, house-sharing, and living in a boarding home.

Specialized housing initiatives frequently have the potential for reshaping an older person's social world at the same time that his or her economic, physical and mental health needs are being attended to. Indeed, a major set of factors influencing the relationship between the elderly and their housing are socially determined. Included here is the trend away from intergenerational living arrangements and the fact that older people move much less frequently than do those of working age (Lawton, 1982). Only about 6 percent of those aged 65 and over move in any one year, which is only about a quarter the rate for adults under the age of 65 (Lawton, 1980). The elderly are also subject to increasing losses in their social and familial networks. This, in turn, affects the quality and quantity of relationships in their environment, the symbolic or affective aspects of their shelter, their feelings of personal security, and their access to services, resources, and social relationships (Sheehan, 1986; American Association of Retired Persons, 1989). The "small-group environment," constituted by family members, networks of friends, neighbors, work colleagues, and similar types of face-to-face aggregates, needs to be considered in any discussion of a particular housing alternative and its relationship to an older person's well-being (Lawton, 1970). The extent to which older residents feel they can exercise some control over their housing environment may also be predictive of their enhanced self-esteem and social involvement (Berkowitz, Waxman, and Yaffe, 1988).

Despite current efforts to improve the living environments of the community aged, several gaps in the knowledge of this subject remain apparent. First, housing alternatives for the frail elderly, as well as the delivery of supportive services in existing housing, should be examined. Such analyses might consider the extent to which service-enriched environments fulfill three central functions of the residential environment — stimulation, maintenance, and support (Lawton, 1989). Furthermore, there has been a clear and unmistakable call for an improvement of and expansion in the range of housing options which: (1) provide a continuum of appropriate alternatives; (2) are located in areas desirable to the elderly; and (3) make use of existing housing stock (White House Conference on Aging, 1981; Katsura, Struyk, and Newman, 1988). In addition to these recommendations there is a need for more research into the improvement of existing housing (Steinfeld, 1981) as well as into innovative enriched housing initiatives for middle income elderly, and not just for low income residents of public housing.

Finally, research is especially needed on the impact that innovative housing initiatives may have on the social lives of elderly tenants as they "age-in" and grow older.

The case study reported here focuses precisely on the latter issue, that is, on the influence that progressive aging may be having on the social lives of elder tenants. It took place at two congregate residences sponsored by a single community agency and inquires into the extent to which the "aging in" process may be related to: (1) patterns of mutual help with other tenants; and (2) patterns of social exchange with relatives and friends who reside outside of the immediate area.

THE STUDY

Data presented are drawn from a sample of elderly tenants (N = 210) residing in two enriched housing facilities sponsored and managed by a voluntary community service organization in New York City: the Jewish Association for Services for the Aged. An 84-item, structured survey instrument was developed and pretested especially for the study and was completed during a person-to-person interview in each respondent's apartment during the winter and spring of 1986. In addition to issues pertaining to social helping patterns, the instrument addressed such topics as: (1) satisfaction with the area and living arrangements; (2) physical and functional health; (3) service knowledge, use, and satisfaction; (4) participation in social activities; (5) life satisfaction; (6) respondent demographics; and (7) resident life events.

A 25 percent random sample of elderly tenants was drawn to participate in the study, resulting in a potential initial N of 356. Two hundred and ten interviews were ultimately performed representing 65 percent of the revised sample (corrected for deceased individuals, those who had moved, and those who were away for the winter or the interview period). The rate of response is considered satisfactory and representative of the larger tenant population given the fact that roughly equal numbers of mobile elderly (those vacationing elsewhere) and those who were either deceased or had moved to more protective environments were ultimately deleted from the initial 25 percent sample.

The study sites represent housing for the elderly with supportive services, following a model of enriched housing. Each was planned to provide fully accessible housing, with appropriate community facilities and supportive social services (Warach, 1986). These two residences, which are situated adjacent to each other in the Rockaway section of New York City, constitute one of the largest congregate, enriched housing projects in the United States. Together they comprise five apartment houses and incorporate a comprehensive senior center. The five buildings were completed over an 18 year period (1967-1985).

A PROFILE OF THE ELDER TENANTS

The vast majority of respondents (95%) were 65 years or older, with more than 6 in 10 respondents (62.7%) over the age of 75. More than half of the respondent group (53.0%) had not gone beyond grammar or grade school education, and most were not engaged in salaried employment. One half indicated they were retired while the remainder categorized their status as unemployed. Only 1 respondent held a part-time job at the time of the study. Residents held a wide variety of former jobs ranging from clerical (21.3%) and laborer positions (21.3%), to managerial/administrative lines (16.7%), and professional or technical careers (10.7%). They less often identified themselves as former crafts, sales, and private household workers.

The average length of residence in the housing complex was 6 years. Eighty-eight percent or 168 respondents were white with an additional 8.9 percent registering as black. The vast majority of participants were female and Jewish. Five out of every 10 persons were widowed (102 or 50%) with an additional 32.8 percent still married. Thirty eight percent indicated birthplaces outside of the United States while an additional 44 percent were born in New York City.

MEASURING THE AVAILABILITY
OF SOCIAL CONFIDANTS

In addition to a series of questions meant to gauge self-reported social exchange patterns and relationships of elder tenants in the housing development, an index measuring the availability of a social confidant was adapted from studies by Ward, Sherman, and Lagory (1984), Cantor (1979), and Wellman (1979). The 5-item "Social Confidant Index" measured the availability of someone to satisfy both expressive needs (talking to someone about a personal problem, someone to share your happiness when you feel good about something) and instrumental needs (someone to help with chores you are unable to do, someone to help when you are sick and in bed, and someone to go to the grocery store when you cannot) along a 4-point Likert-type scale (1 = no, never; 2 = only some of the time; 3 = yes, most of the time; and 4 = yes, all of the time). This index, which proved to be statistically reliable, had a Cronbach's alpha of .82 with a mean of 15.1 and a standard deviation of 4.2. The mean score indicates that, for the most part, respondents had at least one individual available who could be relied on as a social confidant. Respondents were most often found to have someone available to assist them in an expressive need area (i.e., to share in happiness) (mean = 3.3), and least often in an instrumental domain (i.e., help with household chores) (mean = 2.7).

SOCIAL NETWORKS AND THE ELDERLY

This section of survey findings inquired about:

1. the presence of existing social networks of elder residents in the housing complex;
2. the frequency and intensity of contacts between residents and their families, friends, and neighbors; and
3. the types of functions performed by residents and their social networks during periods of need.

Almost 8 of every 10 respondents (79.3%) had living children with 77.4 percent of this group indicating that they had 1 to 3 sons and daughters. Similarly, 73.1 percent of the residents had grandchildren, with 74.4 percent of this group having 6 or fewer grandchildren. The mean number of children and grandchildren for the respondent group was 2.2 and 5.2 respectively. Children were somewhat more likely to live closer to residents than grandchildren and it was usually 1 child rather than 2 who were in close proximity to the older tenant's residence.

Respondents were found to have the most frequent contact with their children, either by telephone or in person, and almost half of those who responded to this question (93 or 49.5%) had contact with their children on a daily basis. Only 1 in 10 (10.1%) respondents had daily contact with their grandchildren. It is worth noting that the vast majority of those surveyed who had relatives maintained at least weekly contact with one or more of their children and grandchildren. On the other hand, 41.4 percent of the respondents indicated that they never spoke to relatives other than children and grandchildren. Only 13.8 and 22.5 percent of respondents admitted to never having contact with their children and grandchildren, respectively.

All relatives, regardless of their position in the family constellation, rarely provided assistance to residents with housekeeping, cooking, and apartment repair. Relatives, especially children, readily assisted during periods of illness. Their help consisted of shopping, errands, giving advice to resolve a problem, providing transportation, and escorting to a doctor. (See Table 1).

Conversely, respondents were found to rarely reciprocate with assistance to relatives. Older residents were more likely to aid their relatives when advice was sought on a particular issue. Even so, only 10 percent of the respondent group ever engaged in such aid. There was an obvious imbalance, as elder residents received more help than they gave to relatives, even though the assistance they got from relatives other than children was quite limited.

Analysis of data confirmed that there was no significant difference in the extent of help received from or provided to children, friends living outside the complex, and other tenants within the complex when considering years of widowhood, tenant self-reported financial status, race/ethnicity, place of birth, level of education and employment status.

Significant difference did emerge, however, when considering religious preference, age, sex, marital status, and years in the housing complex. Specifically, those residents who were not Jewish indicated significantly higher levels of assistance received from their friends who did not live in the housing complex itself. Females were significantly more likely to receive some degree of assistance from their relatives living outside the housing complex than their male counterparts ($\Sigma = 6.02$; df = 3; p < .01). Furthermore, the "old-old," those residents 75 years and older, were significantly less likely to receive assistance and conversely to provide assistance to their community residing friends. Thus, the very cohort of older people who might be expected to need help the most were the least likely to receive it from their friends.

Recent residents displayed significantly higher levels of aid provided to their friends outside the housing complex. These levels decreased over time ($\Sigma = 16.20$; df = 6; p < .01), suggesting in part the growing importance of one's fellow tenants in the mutual aid system at this housing complex, as well as the gradual movement toward more insular relationships among respondents. Finally, single, widowed and divorced/sepa-

TABLE 1. Type and Frequency of Help Received from Relatives Living Outside the Housing Complex

TYPE OF HELP	CHILDREN				GRANDCHILDREN				OTHER RELATIVES			
	SOMETIMES		NEVER		SOMETIMES		NEVER		SOMETIMES		NEVER	
	No.	%	No.	%	No.	%	No.	%	No.	%	No.	%
A. Help out when you are sick	81	44.3	102	55.7	18	11.8	135	88.2	22	15.2	123	84.8
B. Help you with shopping or errands	80	43.0	106	57.0	22	14.9	126	85.1	22	14.9	126	85.1
C. Help you with housecleaning	12	6.5	173	93.5	2	1.3	156	98.7	5	3.3	146	96.7
D. Cook for you	16	8.6	169	91.4	2	1.3	157	98.7	9	6.0	142	94.0
E. Fix things around the apartment	32	17.5	151	82.5	6	3.8	151	96.2	8	5.4	140	94.6
F. Give advice when you have a problem or worry	89	48.6	94	51.4	33	14.6	134	85.4	39	26.9	106	73.1
G. Provide transportation or go with you to the doctor, or social visits, or other places you go	76	41.5	107	58.5	16	10.1	143	89.9	23	15.9	122	84.1

rated respondents claimed higher levels of supportive aid provided to external friends.

Whereas perceived caregiving reciprocity was not evidenced in the case of respondents and their relatives, it was more likely to be reported when considering the nature of relationships between respondents and both their friends outside the housing complex and their on-site tenant neighbors. As shown in Tables 2 and 3, assistance levels were quite similar when comparing the extent of self-reported help received by respondents from friends and tenants, and that provided by respondents.

It is interesting to note that respondents felt that they provided more assistance to their fellow tenants than they received. Such assessments may be expected to vary to some degree depending on the perspective of the respondent (i.e., whether they perceive themselves to be recipients or providers of assistance). Regardless of what may be interpreted as a degree of subjective "distortion" in the respondents' perception of mutual aid, there appeared to be a widespread network of confidant relationships among residents. Two-thirds of the survey group (66.7% or 136) indicated that they had people they felt close to in the building. The mean number of such social confidants per respondent was 4.6.

Respondents were finally asked to identify the person or organization to whom they would turn for help during a personal emergency. Relatives outside the complex and spouses or housemates, should one be present, were identified by tenants as the main line of defense in the eventuality of an emergency (42.9% would turn to such an individual first). Second in acceptance was the housing management office to whom 19.2 percent of the respondents would turn for emergency help. Other residents in the complex, floor captains, police, and social service staff were less frequently reported sources of aid. Community agencies, the clergy, and friends living outside the building were rarely mentioned as sources of help during crises.

SOCIAL SUPPORTS
AND RESPONDENT HEALTH STATUS

The association between measures of social support and indicators of the respondents' health status were examined in a separate correlational analysis (see Table 4). It was found that those residents who reported they were in better health provided more assistance to relatives ($r = .17$; $p < .01$) and received more frequent assistance from neighbors living outside the building ($r = .15$; $p < .05$), while those in poorer health experienced less frequent contact with their externally-situated social support network

TABLE 2. Self-Reported Help Received from Friends and Provided to Friends by Respondents

TYPE OF HELP	RECEIVED FROM FRIENDS				GIVEN TO FRIENDS			
	Yes		No		Yes		No	
	No.	%	No.	%	No.	%	No.	%
A. Help when sick	29	23.4	95	76.6	34	27.6	89	72.4
B. Help with shopping or errands	31	25.0	93	75.0	27	22.0	96	78.0
C. Help with housecleaning	6	4.8	118	95.2	5	4.1	118	95.9
D. Cooking	14	11.4	109	88.6	11	9.0	111	91.0
E. Fixing things around the apartment	14	11.4	109	88.6	11	8.9	112	91.1
F. Giving advice for a problem or worrying	49	39.5	75	60.5	50	41.0	72	59.0
G. Providing transportation or going to the doctor, or social visits, or other places	50	41.0	72	59.0	23	18.9	99	81.1

TABLE 3. Self-Reported Help Received from and Provided to Fellow Tenants by Respondents

TYPES OF ASSISTANCE*	RECEIVED FROM TENANTS				GIVEN TO TENANTS			
	Yes		No		Yes		No	
	No.	%	No.	%	No.	%	No.	%
A. Looking in to see how one is doing	121	59.0	84	41.0	127	62.0	78	38.0
B. Going with you/them to the doctor, shopping, etc.	33	16.1	172	83.9	47	22.9	158	77.1
C. Getting things for you/them at the store	54	26.3	151	73.7	72	35.1	133	64.9
D. Talking to you/them about personal concerns and problems	70	34.1	135	65.9	91	44.4	114	55.6
E. Looking after the apartment when you/they are away	41	20.0	164	80.0	42	20.6	162	79.4
F. Lending you/them things (other than money)	29	14.1	176	85.9	49	24.0	155	76.0
G. Helping you/them in case of an emergency	54	26.3	151	73.7	96	47.1	108	52.9

*Assistance provided/received during the past 12 months.

TABLE 4. Pearson's Correlations Between Measures of Social Support and Health Status

Social Support Measures	Self-Reported Health	Number of Days Sick in Last 6 Months	Functional Health Status
Frequency of Assistance Provided to Relatives	.17**	-.09	-.01
Frequency of Assistance Provided to Friends	.08	-.09	-.13*
Frequency of Assistance Received from Neighbors	.15*	-.08	-.26***
Frequency of Contact with Social Support Network	-.14*	.08	.04
Size of Social Support Network	.09	-.16*	-.21**
Number of Social Confidents	.07	-.18**	-.08

* $p < .05$
** $p < .01$
*** $p < .001$

($r = -.14$; $p < .05$). Similarly, the more days they were sick, the less likely respondents were to report having a social confidant ($r = -.18$; $p < .01$), and the more circumscribed their external social support network ($r = -.16$; $p < .05$). Similar results were found when considering functional health status. While the correlations were relatively weak, findings nevertheless revealed that declining respondent functional health status was associated with declining size of one's external social support network ($r = -.21$; $p < .01$), as well as reductions in support received from fellow tenants ($r = -.26$; $p < .001$). Thus, those elders with presumably the greatest degree of need appear to have received the least assistance and support. These findings are similar to those obtained by Stephens, Kinney, and McNeer (1986), which document greater degrees of social isolation or separation on the parts of the functionally impaired in a life care facility.

LIFE SATISFACTION AND SOCIAL RELATIONS

The strength of the respondents social support networks was associated with their personal sense of life satisfaction. The life satisfaction measure was based on the combined responses to 4 items adapted from the Duke University OARS questionnaire (Pfeiffer, 1976); the frequency of feelings of loneliness, the degree of worry over life events, the level of excitement in one's life, and a general assessment of satisfaction with life at the present time. Findings confirmed that as the number of available social supports increases (e.g., children, grandchildren, other relatives, friends and fellow tenants) satisfaction with life increases ($r = .22$; $p < .01$). Furthermore, increments in the amount of self-reported help provided by respondents to externally residing friends was positively associated with heightened life satisfaction ($r = .14$; $p < .05$). Interestingly, the reverse was not the case, that is, increased help provided by friends living outside the complex was not correlated with increments in expressed contentment. This suggests that the opportunity to help others is more satisfying than the experience of receiving help.

Other data served to reaffirm the relationship between contentment and health. Contentment, as measured by the index of life satisfaction, was negatively associated with the number of sick days that respondents had experienced in the past six months ($r = -.27$; $p < .001$). Heightened levels of contentment were positively associated with respondents' self assessments of their overall health ($r = .35$; $p < .001$).

SUMMARY AND CONCLUSIONS

This single site study made use of a series of subjective as well as objective measures of the housing environment in order to arrive at a better understanding of the social exchange patterns of older adults residing in urban-based enriched housing. Subjective indicators have been previously recognized as positive methodological tools for gaining insight into the housing status of older Americans (Golant, 1986). Enriched housing respondents participating in this analysis were found to maintain intense family relationships with their children, although these ties tended to weaken with age. Tenant interactions with grandchildren and other relatives (i.e., siblings, nieces, and nephews) were substantially less intense than those sustained with their offspring.

A lack of symmetry would appear present in terms of perceived assistance exchanges between residents and other relatives. Kin were significantly more likely to provide assistance to respondents with various activities of daily living than the reverse. On the other hand, self-reported exchange symmetry did emerge in reference to externally residing friends and fellow tenants. The frequency and intensity of exchanges with community dwelling friends reached higher levels than those between respondents and their relatives living outside the complex. Female residents received higher levels of assistance as compared to males. The same was true for the young-old compared to those 75 years of age and over. Gaps in social support networks were closely associated with decrements recorded in personal contentment with one's situation.

Drawing implications from these data to the larger congregate housing field should only cautiously be undertaken as this was a case study restricted to two adjoining housing sites in the New York City metropolitan area. Comparative data on alternative housing programs elsewhere in the country were not offered. In addition, while the protocol developed for this study was submitted to systematic pretesting, selected measures were utilized for the first time in this research and could thus benefit from additional test administrations on elder populations in other congregate settings. Furthermore, this was a cross-sectional study which limited data collection to a single point in time rather than performing repeated measures over an extended period in the lives of the respondents. Yet, the findings about the relationship between social support networks on the one hand, and age and life satisfaction on the other, are regarded to be of importance for future planning and programming.

As the "aging in" process inevitably progresses, enriched housing programs, such as the one studied in this research, may be pressed to think about initiating specialized programs which aim to rectify or improve poorly balanced relations between frail community elders and their external informal support systems. The Housing administrators may also want to consider the benefits of promoting accommodating or flexible, as compared to constant, environments (as conceptualized by Lawton, 1980, 1985). This could be accomplished in part be encouraging the participation of informal network support services as well as other more commonly offered social and health services.

Neglecting natural helping networks in specialized housing may have costly consequences. Enriched housing administrators may be compelled to either arrange for the premature relocation of frail elder tenants or deliver exceedingly intense and costly health and social services to these individuals simply because the elder's helping network has prematurely shrunk or disintegrated altogether. Early intervention in the form of housing policies and programs that promote social exchange and support between older tenants and their significant others, both within and outside of the housing development, may ultimately ensure increasingly satisfying lives for the elderly themselves at the same time that the costs of extending formal services can be kept at bay.

REFERENCES

American Association of Retired Persons. (1989). Studies explore service needs of elderly public housing residents. *AARP Housing Report,* 1-3.

Berkowitz, M.W., Waxman, R., and Yaffe, L. (1988). The effects of a resident self-help model on control, social involvement and self-esteem among the elderly. *The Gerontologist,* 28, 620-624.

Cantor, M. (1979). Neighbors and friends: An overlooked resource in the informal support system. *Research on Aging,* 1, 434-463.

Carp, F.M. (1976). Housing and living environments of older people. In Binstock, R.H. and Shanas, E. (Eds.). *Handbook of Aging and the Social Sciences.* New York: Van Nostrand Reinhold, Inc.

Golant, S.M. (1986). Subjective housing assessments by the elderly: A critical information source for planning and program evaluation. *The Gerontologist,* 26, 122-127.

Hinrichsen, G.A. (1985). The impact of age-concentrated, publicly assisted housing on older people's social and emotional well-being. *Journal of Gerontology,* 40, 758-760.

Katsura, H.M., Struyk, R.J., and Newman, S.J. (1988). *Housing for the Elderly in 2010: Projections and Policy Options.* Washington, DC: The Urban Institute.

Lawton, M.P. (1970). Ecology and aging. In Pastalan, L.A. and Carson, D.H.

(Eds.). *Special Behavior of Older People*. Ann Arbor, MI: Institute of Gerontology, University of Michigan.

Lawton, M.P. (1980). *Environment and Aging*. Monterey, CA: Brooks/Cole.

Lawton, M.P. (1982). Environments and living arrangements. In Binstock, R.H., Chow, W., and Schulz, J.H. (Eds.). *International Perspectives on Aging: Population and Policy Challenges*. New York: United Nations Fund for Population Activities.

Lawton, M.P. (1985). Housing and living environments of older people. In Binstock, R.H. and Shanas, E. (Eds.). *Handbook of Aging and the Social Sciences*. New York, N.Y.: Van Nostrand Reinhold Company, Inc.

Lawton, M.P. (1989). Three functions of the residential environment. In Pastalan, L.A., and Cowart, M.E. (Eds.). *Lifestyles and Housing of Older Adults: The Florida Experience*. New York, NY: The Haworth Press, Inc.

Lawton, M.P. and Cohen, J. (1974). The generality of housing impact on the well being of older people. *Journal of Gerontology*, 29, 194-204.

Pfeiffer, E. (Ed.). (1976). *Multidimensional Functional Assessment: The OARS Methodology*. Durham, N.C.: Center for the Study of Aging and Human Development.

Select Committee on Aging, House of Representatives. (1988). *Dignity, Independence, and Cost Effectiveness: The Success of the Congregate Housing Services Program*. Washington, DC: U.S. Government Printing Office. (Comm. Pub. No. 100-670).

Sheehan, N.W. (1986). Informal support among the elderly in public senior housing. *The Gerontologist*. 26, 171-175.

Sherman, S.R. (1985). Housing. In Monk, A. (Ed.). *Handbook of Gerontological Services*. New York, N.Y.: Van Nostrand Reinhold Company, Inc.

Sherwood, S., Greer, D.S., and Morris, J.N. (1979). A study of the highland heights apartments for the physically impaired and elderly in Fall River. In Byerts, T.O., Howell, S.C., and Pastalan, L.A. (Eds.). *Environmental Context of Aging*. New York: Garland STPM Press.

Steinfeld, E. (1981). The scope of residential repair and renovation services and models of service delivery. In Lawton, M.P. and Hoover, S.L. (Eds.). *Community Housing Choices for Older Americans*. New York: Springer Publishing Company.

Stephens, M.A.P., Kinney, J.M., and McNeer, A.E. (1986). Accommodative housing: Social integration of residents with physical limitations. *The Gerontologist*, 26, 176-180.

Turner, L. and Magnum, E. (1982). Report of the Housing Choices of Older Americans: Executive Summary." Final report submitted to the Administration on Aging, Office of Human Development Services, U.S. Department of Health and Human Services. (Grant No. 90-AR-2118).

Warach, B. (1986). Supportive services in housing for the elderly: emerging needs and problems, *Journal of Jewish Communal Service*, 62, 299-306.

Ward, R.A., Sherman, S.R., and LaGory, M. (1984). Subjective network assessments and subjective well-being. *Journal of Gerontology,* 39, 93-101.

Wellman, B. (1979). The community question: The intimate networks of East Yorkers. *American Journal of Sociology*, 84, 1201-1231.

White House Conference on Aging. (1981). *Report of the Mini-Conference on Housing for the Elderly.* Washington, DC: U.S. Government Printing Office. (Publication #1981 720-019/6916).

The Design of Supportive Environments for Older People

Michael E. Hunt

INTRODUCTION

The goal of designing a supportive environment is to maximize a person's competence or ability to function within an environment, whether it be a building, a neighborhood or a city. Environmental competence is a function of two components: someone's personal capabilities and the characteristics of the environment itself. Thus, it is highly unlikely that one could design a supportive environment without first understanding the needs and capabilities of the inhabitants. The environment can then be designed to accommodate the person rather than expecting that the person will adapt to the environment.

The concepts of supportive environments and environmental competence are useful for two main reasons. First, they help dispel the notion that supportive design results from following a list of prescribed environmental attributes assumed to be essential for older residents. Supportive design is, after all, a goal, not merely the successful implementation of a list of physical attributes. Second, these concepts help place design in the larger context of the total environment – in this case, the total living environment of congregate housing. Two examples illustrate this important point.

Michael E. Hunt, ArchD, is Associate Director of the Institute on Aging and Adult Life, and Associate Professor in the Environment, Textiles and Design Department at the University of Wisconsin-Madison. His duties at the University of Wisconsin include administering the educational programs of the Institute on Aging and teaching and conducting research in the areas of housing for older people, environment and behavior studies, and building evaluation. He has co-authored a book on retirement communities and has written articles concerning housing for older people and environmental learning.

HOW TO DESIGN A NON-PERSON

An excellent example of why environmental design must be considered in the larger context of the total living environment is an audiotape entitled *How To Design a Non-Person* (no date, Institute of Gerontology, University of Michigan). The message is made especially poignant by being presented as a satire. Four categories of methods for designing a non-person are presented.

1. Confuse her. Start this by moving her from a familiar environment to an unfamiliar one and locate the housing in an unfamiliar neighborhood where she will feel lost. Design the housing so that it is out of touch with the outdoors to lose the sense of seasons and limit natural daylight, so that she also loses a sense of time of day. Destroy the clues to spaces she inhabits by using long corridors and repeating the same elements endlessly such as doors, windows, furniture, colors, and textures.

2. Take away her identity. Remove her private telephone by using a switchboard. This will remove her name from the telephone directory, and people will eventually give up trying to locate her. Long-distance calls will need to be the more expensive person-to-person and thus shorter and less frequent. Take away her self-identity by furnishing her apartment with furniture identical to all other apartments, limit her possessions to a minimum, and omit pin-up space for mementos. Modify her self-image by referring to her as a patient rather than a resident and use large undifferentiated spaces with high ceilings to make her feel small and unimportant.

3. Make her dependent and submissive with no will power. Don't allow her into the decision-making process. Make rules for her and post them in hallways and inside apartment doors. Utilize her disabilities to keep her dependent by using round doorknobs instead of lever handles on doors, and locate light switches, electrical outlets, and storage shelves just out of reach. Provide low seating that is inconvenient when rising and use heavy glass doors that are difficult to maneuver with a cane or walker and impossible in a wheelchair.

4. Reduce her social contacts. Isolate her by placing her in the country or in the suburbs on the edge of town. Limit contacts with family and friends by regulating visiting hours and providing large impersonal lounges shared by others. Don't provide places to share food during family gatherings, or places to entertain children and grandchildren. In public lounges and dining areas, use formal furniture positioned to avoid small groupings and eye contact. This way the family member will acquire the role of visitor rather than relative.

These examples taken from the audiotape in reference illustrate how similar situations that occur all too often for the sake of older people involve the total living environment including design and administration. The examples also show that failing to achieve supportiveness in one part of the total environment diminishes the success of another.

NATURALLY OCCURRING RETIREMENT COMMUNITIES

A second example of why environmental design must be considered in the larger context of the total living environment is provided by naturally occurring retirement communities. A naturally occurring retirement community (NORC) is defined as housing or a residential area not planned or designed for older people, but which attracts a preponderance of older residents (Hunt & Gunter-Hunt, 1986). NORCs are an interesting housing option because they have attracted older residents without the benefit of specialized advertising, age segregation, payment subsidies, or health related services. It is important to understand what has naturally attracted older residents to NORCs in order to plan and design the attractive attributes of NORCs into congregate housing.

Hunt's study (1988) of the attractions of NORC apartment complexes found three main categories of factors involved in the evolution of a NORC: (1) location; (2) management; and (3) design. Location seems to be the initial attraction of a NORC for older residents. There are two main aspects of location that appear to be important: (1) most importantly, proximity to friends and family; and (2) proximity to shopping and amenities. Management was found to be critical in maintaining a stream of referrals to the NORC. Since NORC older residents seem to expect and even demand that the NORC be well maintained and since most NORC older residents were attracted to the NORC by word-of-mouth, it appears that management plays a key role in fostering the evolution of a NORC. Finally, the design of a NORC does not seem to be an attraction, but rather a potential barrier to continued independent living. Thus, design is an important aspect of the NORC appeal, but it is certainly not sufficient unto itself.

This insight into what attracts older people to housing not planned or designed for them, and in fact sometimes poorly designed for them, illustrates that a person's attraction to housing is a multifaceted construct that entails the collaboration of those involved in planning and administering as well as designing the housing.

SUPPORTIVE ENVIRONMENTS
FOR OLDER RESIDENTS

To discuss the design of supportive housing for older residents, it is helpful to establish an organizational framework from which to address such a broad subject. The framework is attractive because it addresses the design of supportive environments from the perspective of older residents themselves.

As stated above, a supportive environment is one that meets the needs and capabilities of its inhabitants. In the framework, people's needs and capabilities are divided into three categories: (1) physical needs; (2) informational needs; and (3) social needs.

Physical Needs

A person's physical needs are those that involve sustaining acceptable physical health and comfort levels. This perhaps is the first subject that comes to mind when thinking of designing for older people. However, care should be taken not to succumb to the convenient notion that the goal is to design for a handicapped individual. Rather, the goal is to design for a person who prefers and possibly needs a residence that is convenient and easy to maintain because, due to the normal aging process, the older person is not as able to compensate for poorly designed housing as effectively as in the past. Leonard has referred to such places as handicapped buildings (1978).

An excellent example of supportive housing is Orange Gardens in Kissimmee, Florida. Interestingly, Orange Gardens is not new, having opened in 1955. According to its developer, it has the distinction of being the first subdivision in the country to be architecturally designed for retirement living. However, it was also planned that 15 to 20 percent of the residents should be younger families, some of which would have young children in the household.

All of the over 500 homes in Orange Gardens were especially designed for older residents. The homes were built barrier-free, inside and outside. In addition, the kitchen and bathrooms were specially equipped because these are the areas in the home where most accidents occur. In the kitchen, cabinets were mounted to minimize climbing and stooping. In the bathroom, all fixtures were bolted to wall studs for support. Handholds were mounted around the end and side of the tub and behind the toilet. Even the soap dishes and shower-curtain rods were reinforced. With the reinforcement provided, all of these fixtures could support up to 1,000 pounds. Thus a person could grab any of the fixtures for support. The toilet was also placed next to the bathtub in order to help the person get into the tub. With this positioning, a person could sit on the toilet, then swing her legs into the tub, and then shift her body into the tub. The tubs were also equipped with non-skid strips.

There were other special features in the houses as well. All electric outlets were placed 26 inches above the floor to minimize stooping. Baseboards were dark to provide contrast between the floor plane and the wall plane. And finally, all doors were made wide enough to admit a wheelchair.

A potential danger of designing homes especially for older people is that they might not attract the younger residents, who were to represent 15 to 20 percent of Orange Gardens' population. However, this problem never developed. There were even two homes designed specifically for paraplegic residents. For example, no cabinets were placed under the sinks to allow for wheelchair access. When these homes were resold, the new owners never realized that they were specialized homes. Likewise, the resale of other homes in Orange Gardens has never been a problem because of the special design features for older people. Instead, Orange Gardens' reputation has evolved into one of a high quality subdivision— not a retirement community. Thus, the Orange Gardens experience indicates that housing that is supportive of and attractive to older people is attractive to younger people as well. For more information on Orange Gardens, see Hunt et al., (1984).

Other design features that address a person's physical needs include furniture selection, the lowering of windows to enable seated residents to enjoy viewing outdoors, the design of stairs should they be necessary, and flooring materials. In the above referenced NORC research, it was learned that inconvenient access to laundry facilities, trash receptacles, mail boxes, and auto parking presented potential barriers to older residents' continued independent living in apartment complexes. Two excellent books that address the physical needs of older people in addition to other related subjects are Raschko (1982) and the American Institute of Architects (1985).

Informational Needs

A person's informational needs concern how information about the environment and other people is processed. Two main aspects of information processing should be addressed: perception and cognition. Perception is the process of obtaining or receiving environmental information. Cognition is discussed from the perspective of how people organize and remember environmental information. Together, perception and cognition make up an information processing system that must be addressed by environmental design if a given environment is to support the needs and capabilities of its inhabitants.

Perception

The perceptual needs and capabilities of older people are important to address when designing supportive housing because an aging person experiences normal and irreversible sensory changes. Changes occur in vision, hearing, touch, taste, and smell that are not related to accident or disease.

The decline in vision with age results from changes in the eye itself. The lens of the eye becomes increasingly rigid and opaque and also gradually yellows. In addition, the surrounding eye muscles begin to weaken and become more lax. As a result of these physical changes, older people experience decreases in their abilities to see objects clearly, focus on objects at different distances, function in low light levels, discern certain color intensities, and judge distances.

The hearing loss that results from normal aging is termed presbycusis. Presbycusis is a progressive loss of hearing, although the symptoms are not usually apparent until a person is over 65 years of age. The effects of presbycusis generally are two-fold: (1) the inability to hear high frequencies; and (2) the reduced ability to hear sounds in general. As a result, speech may sound garbled, muffled, and difficult to understand.

For an environment to be supportive of older people, it must address these sensory declines. The goal is to maximize the perceptual capabilities of older residents and help them to compensate for sensory losses by sensorially enriching the housing. Failure to do so makes it increasingly difficult for a resident to adequately perceive the environment around them.

One method for supporting perceptual needs is termed "redundant cuing," which means to provide the environmental message through more than one sensory modality. In this way, the message has a better chance of being perceived because one sensory modality helps to compensate for another. For example, a change in color may be accompanied by a change in texture. This example can be utilized on flooring to warn of level changes such as stairs or ramps or on wall surfaces to help identify or distinguish different spaces. It should be noted that this is no different than providing a warning track for outfielders in baseball to warn them of the outfield wall. Texture can even be added to handrails to alert people to the beginning and ending of stairways since most stair accidents occur at the top or bottom of the stairway.

Other examples of redundant cuing include designing to allow sound and smell to supplement vision. For example, design the common dining areas in such a way that the sound and aroma are allowed to permeate the nearby areas and serve as environmental cues and possibly enticements to enter. Similarly the sounds of activity in nearby game, craft, or patio areas can serve as environmental cues as well as enticements. Using such redundant cuing as an enticement to enter has not gone unnoticed by retailers such as bakeries that allow the aroma of their wares to drift out onto the sidewalk or into the mall and lure in unsuspecting customers.

The design of supportive environments for older residents also addresses several specific types of sensory loss. For example, it is estimated that an 80-year-old person needs about three times more light to read a book than that needed by a teenager. However, older people also experience an exaggerated amount of glare from an intense light source. Thus, an older person is further hindered by merely using stronger light sources to increase the light level. Rather, multiple sources of indirect lighting should be used while avoiding glossy finishes on floors and walls. Extreme changes in illumination level should be avoided as well.

Difficulty in discerning color intensities results from the yellowing of the lens of the eye. Colors particularly affected are in the blue and green sector of the color spectrum. This does not imply that blue and green colors should be avoided. Rather, the implication is to avoid using these colors adjacent to each other unless higher intensity varieties of the colors are used.

To help older residents see planar differences, adjoining planes, such as a wall and a floor, should be colored distinctively to accentuate the intersection.

The declining ability to hear resulting from presbycusis can also be addressed by environmental design. For example, background noises should be avoided, and furniture should be arranged in small clusters allowing eye contact to permit the reading of lips.

For a more thorough discussion of designing to compensate for vision and hearing impairments, see Hiatt (1987).

Cognition

As stated above, cognition is discussed from the perspective of how people organize and remember environmental information. In this regard, the goal of environmental design is to design buildings that are understandable or imageable. This can be addressed from two perspectives: (1) designing an imageable building; and (2) helping residents learn the building, regardless of its inherent imageability.

Imageable Design. Weisman (1987) has identified four classes of architectural attributes that maximize the imageability of a building. First is the category of signs and numbers which are the identification and directional information supplied in a building. Architectural differentiation is the second category that is defined as the distinctiveness of various elements or regions in the building. Perceptual access is the third category and refers to the resident's ability to perceive a destination through one or more sensory modalities before actually arriving there. The final category is plan configuration that refers to an understanding of the basic configuration of the building.

Signs and numbers are the most common wayfinding cues in buildings and should be designed to augment the information provided by the environment. To aid perception, signs generally should consist of light letters on a dark background. The location of signs is also an important consideration. Identification signs should be placed on the wall next to the door on the door handle side. This way the sign can be read when the door is open. Signs identifying especially important places should be mounted perpendicular to the wall so as to be read from down a hallway. Direction signs should be carefully positioned as well. They should be at major hallway intersections, opposite elevators, and in public waiting areas. Signs can even be color-coded to reflect regional color differentiations in the building.

The architectural attribute of perceptual access is based on the notion that it is easier to find a destination if it can be seen, heard, smelled, or perceived in any way prior to arrival there. One way to accomplish this goal is to make it possible to see into a room or smell or hear it, before actually entering. Then, the resident can decide if entering is desirable or may even be drawn into the space. Another way to utilize this design attribute is to provide views to the outside. Such views help to relate the resident's position to the outside and to the building as a whole. A third way is to provide views to other parts of the building's interior. This is often accomplished by using atriums or courtyards.

Architectural differentiation refers to the need for variety in a building to help residents recognize their relative location. Depending upon the scale being considered, differentiation can result in landmarks or identifiable districts within a building. Landmarks can be virtually any identifiable element in the building: art work, furniture, a window view, or a place such as a dining room. Thus, care should be taken to avoid monotonous color, texture, and furniture selection. Particular places in the buildings should be identifiable as well. Room entrances, views off elevators, and corridor intersections are but a few examples. Regions or districts of the building should also be designed with variety. Corridor segments and other functional areas such as recreation, dining, public, and residential should be differentiated.

An appropriate analogy to this design attribute is the residential area where the residents lived previously. Not every house, street, or neighborhood looked alike. That variety helped them and others find and identify their home. All too often, housing designed for older people is the most environmentally sterile and unstimulating place in which the older resident has ever lived. Ironically, this occurs just at a time when the older person may need or appreciate an environment that is more, not less, supportive of their needs and capabilities.

Plan configuration is the final architectural attribute identified by Weisman that aids in understanding a building. It refers to an understanding of the spatial relationships within the building. Interestingly, an understanding of plan configuration can be maximized by adequately addressing the first three architectural attributes interactively. For example, plan sign systems to reflect color coding of districts, use perceptual access to reveal architectural differentiation in other parts of the building as well as plan configuration, and use signs to help teach the building's plan configuration. Clearly, these four architectural attributes need to be thought of as a system in which one attribute presents and reinforces the others.

Environmental Learning. As important as it is to design imageable buildings, it may not be sufficient to help a resident understand the building. It is also important to provide an environmental learning technique to help residents learn the building, regardless of its inherent imageability.

An environmental learning technique that helps older people has been developed and successfully evaluated (Hunt, 1985; Hunt & Pastalan, 1987; Hunt & Roll, 1987). The technique was based on the two essential types of information needed to formulate an understanding of a building: identification and spatial orientation. An early version of the technique was composed of a schematic architectural model of the building's interior and a series of sequential photographic slides. A later version of the technique was composed of an oblique drawing of the building's interior and a few photographs of key elements in the building. Both versions were found to familiarize older people with an unknown building at least as well as taking an actual visit to the building. In addition, the architecture model was found useful in orienting visually impaired residents to the building.

An environmental learning technique can serve at least two functions. First, it can help reduce stress resulting from relocation to the housing by helping the new resident learn and understand the building even before the move takes place. Second, incorporating the technique into the building's signage system can reinforce the resident's understanding of the building and aid in wayfinding.

Social Needs

A person's social needs are those that pertain to achieving desired levels of social interaction. Meeting the resident's social needs implies empowering residents with control over the environment and their lives. This seems especially important in the context of housing for older people since residents have lived most of their lives in houses where they had ownership and complete social control. They had places that were distinctively their own, other places primarily for family, others for interacting with friends, and still others, such as a front porch, where they could watch outsiders and even interact with them if so desired while still remaining on their turf—their home. To leave such social control and move to congregate housing where all too often social control is lost is a difficult transition. At risk is the loss of a feeling of being at home only to be replaced by a feeling of being a resident in housing for the elderly.

Meeting social needs must be addressed at three overlapping levels. The first concerns the ambiance of the housing. How can it be designed to feel like home even though it has none of the family history, emotional significance and memories of the home left behind? Second is fostering a sense of community within the congregate housing. How can environmental design foster a sense of camaraderie and belonging among residents? Finally, the congregate housing should be linked with the surrounding community. How can environmental design facilitate interaction among residents of congregate housing and the surrounding neighborhood?

The Ambiance

The ambiance of congregate housing should be home-like. It should look and feel residential, not institutional. To help accomplish this goal, the building(s) should be designed to blend in to the surrounding neighborhood—to be a good neighbor aesthetically. Typical design characteristics of the surrounding neighborhood could be integrated into the congregate housing design—e.g., roof style, building materials, architectural style, and even window style. In this way, the congregate housing embodies some of the characteristics associated with what is familiar. Interior lighting and furniture selection are also important in the ambiance of housing. There should be variety in both, and care should be taken to minimize the use of fluorescent lighting and to avoid the use of institutional-looking furniture. In public areas, furniture should be placed in small groupings, and large open undifferentiated spaces should be avoided. Wall and flooring surface materials and window treatments should also be homey as well as easy to maintain.

Design should also allow residents to feel as though their individual apartment reflects their personality and the very essence of themselves. Residents should be allowed to furnish their own apartment, and it should be designed to allow multiple furniture arrangements. There should be generous wall and shelf space for pictures and mementos. The apartment should also be designed to permit entertaining a small number of friends. This can be accomplished by providing a kitchen and dining space with the kitchen designed to allow conversation with people in the living room. Backstage areas such as the bedroom and bathroom should be kept distinct from the more public areas of the apartment. The door to the apartment should allow personalization as well. For example, a tackable surface could be placed next to the door permitting the display of an item identifying the resident.

The living space of the apartment should also reach beyond the walls of the apartment unit itself. This can be accomplished with a patio or balcony as well as a form of front porch. Front porches are wonderful vehicles for neighboring while staying at home and can be designed by simply recessing the hallway wall near the apartment door to create a wide spot in the hall large enough to permit the placement of a porch chair. A window out to the porch area of the hallway is another innovative way to link the apartment to the hallway community.

Fostering a Sense of Community

The key to fostering a sense of community is to provide places where neighboring can occur naturally. Neighboring tends to occur in transition spaces such as major entry ways and in places where people are attracted on a regular basis such as mailboxes, laundry facilities, congregate dining areas, entrances to the building, and a person's hallway or neighborhood.

Corridor segments can become more than just circulation space with the addition of front porches to apartments as suggested above. Residents can sit on the porch or even see out the front window, as suggested above, and see neighbors come and go and foster chance meetings and conversations. This also permits a constant surveillance of the building which fosters a sense of security and social control.

The entrance to the congregate dining room should contain a lounge with small furniture groupings to permit chance and planned encounters before and after meals. Similarly, a lounge should be placed near the mailboxes so that residents have a place to sit and read mail, talk to each other and proudly display the occasional picture of a grandchild. Dining and receiving mail are two important times in the day, and the building should be designed so that residents can enjoy them to the fullest.

The building's main entrance is another popular spot with residents. Sitting there allows residents to keep tabs on what is happening in the building, and the entry lounge should reflect this important role. It should be a place where residents can stop and talk on their way in and out and a place where administration and residents can routinely interact.

Activity spaces in the building should be clustered and located in convenient and desirable areas of the building. Generous seating in small clusters should be present in all activity areas and service areas. Such seating, for example, can be located near the laundry room to permit neighboring while doing the laundry. However, the location of laundry rooms should not impose unwanted social encounters or place one's laundry on display.

For a more complete discussion of the subject, see Hoglund (1985).

Linking with the Neighborhood

Linking congregate housing with the neighborhood helps maximize resident involvement in the larger community and helps residents not to feel isolated in housing for the elderly. Involvement with the neighborhood may take the form of frequent outings or merely observation, but is important nevertheless.

Observation of the surrounding areas can be accommodated by designing spaces that place residents outside the boundaries of the building, yet inside, such as porches and patios. These places can also be extensions of interior spaces such as lobbies or lounges.

To encourage outings into the neighborhood, the congregate housing must be located near attractive locales such as a neighborhood mall, a library, coffee shop, or any place that conveniently permits being among people. People love to watch people.

Some attempts have been made to link congregate housing with the neighborhood by attracting neighborhood residents into the congregate housing. This could be accomplished by offering adult or child day care or by opening a coffee shop or snack area for use by neighborhood residents. These more aggressive approaches illustrate that linkages between congregate housing and the neighborhood can, and perhaps should, occur in both directions.

CONCLUSION

One of the desirable features of addressing the design of congregate housing from the supportive environment perspective is that it places the older residents at the heart of the subject. Design is considered in terms of how it can unobtrusively support the needs and capabilities of older people, their life situation, their wants and expectations. One of the interesting outcomes of this approach is the realization that every design goal and suggested solution posited above supports not only older people, but the younger of us too. Hence the conclusion that supportive housing for older people is in fact just good housing — for all of us.

REFERENCES

American Institute of Architects (1985). *Design for aging: An architect's guide.* Washington, DC: The AIA Press.

Hoglund, D. J. (1985). *Housing for the elderly: Privacy and independence in environments for the aging.* New York: Van Nostrand Reinhold.

Hiatt, L. G. (1987). Designing for the vision and hearing impairments of the elderly. In V. Regnier and J. Pynoos (Eds.), *Housing the aged: Design directives and policy consideration* (pp. 341-372). New York: Elsevier.

Hunt, M. E. (1984). Environmental learning without being there. *Environment and Behavior, 16*(3), 307-334.

Hunt, M. E. (1985). Enhancing a building's imageability. *Journal of Architectural and Planning Research, 2,* 151-168.

Hunt, M. E. (1988). Transition over time: The naturally occurring retirement community. In G. Gutman and N. Blackie (Eds.), *Housing the very old* (pp. 161-172). Burnaby, British Columbia: Gerontology Research Center, Simon Fraser University.

Hunt, M. E., Feldt., A. G., Marans, R. W., Pastalan, L. A., & Vakalo, K. L. (1984). *Retirement communities: An American original.* New York: The Haworth Press, Inc.

Hunt, M. E., & Gunter-Hunt, G. (1986). Naturally occurring retirement communities. *Journal of Housing for the Elderly, 3*(3), 3-21.

Hunt, M. E., & Pastalan, L. A. (1987). Easing relocation: An environmental learning process. In V. Regnier and J. Pynoos (Eds.), *Housing the aged: Design directives and policy consideration* (pp. 421-440). New York: Elsevier.

Hunt, M. E., & Roll, M. K. (1987). Simulation in familiarizing older people with an unknown building. *The Gerontologist, 27*(2), 169-175.

Institute of Gerontology, University of Michigan (no date). *How to design a nonperson.* An audiotape. Ann Arbor.

Leonard, E. (1978). The handicapped building. *Rehabilitation Literature, 39*(9), 265-269.

Raschko, B. B. (1982). *Housing interiors for the disabled and elderly*. New York: Van Nostrand Reinhold.

Weisman, G. D. (1987). Improving way-finding and architectural legibility in housing for the elderly. In V. Regnier and J. Pynoos (Eds.), *Housing the aged: Design directives and policy consideration* (pp. 441-464). New York: Elsevier.

Enriched Housing for the Elderly: The JASA Experience (1968-1990)

Bernard Warach

The Jewish Association for Services for the Aged (JASA) was organized in 1968 by the Federation of Jewish Philanthropies of New York to provide comprehensive social services and housing facilities for the elderly of New York City, Nassau and Suffolk Counties. Its primary mission was to fill unmet needs of the elderly through programs that could assist the aged to maintain their own lives in their own homes with dignity and autonomy.

Today JASA and its subsidiary home care and housing agencies serve 62,500 elderly over 60 years of age, through a network of local social service offices, senior centers, home care programs, apartment houses, legal services, and its Joint Public Affairs Committee. These services are funded at an annual cost in FY 1989-90 of $62 million by the federal, state and local governments, fees and rents of elderly beneficiaries, grants from the United Jewish Appeal-Federation of Jewish Philanthropies of New York, Board contributions, and other philanthropic sources.

The development and management of housing for the elderly with support services — "enriched housing" — was a central objective from the outset. The plight of thousands of poor aged, residing in deteriorating crime-ridden neighborhoods, in walk-up tenements, isolated and fearful, was compelling testimony to the need for relocation to enriched housing.

JASA'S lay and professional leadership had the opportunity to consider

Bernard Warach, MSW, is Executive Vice President of the Jewish Association for Services for the Aged. He is a former executive of the Associated YM-YWHA's of Greater New York, the Irene Kaufmann Settlement House, the International Refugee Organization, and the U.N. Relief and Rehabilitation Administration. Mr. Warach is a lecturer in schools of social work and a Fellow of the Gerontological Society of America.

in depth the varied models in development of housing for the elderly with supporting services. By 1968 some notable housing for the aged facilities had been completed in New York City and throughout the nation. One enriched housing model, incorporated into the development of Kittay House, sponsored by Jewish Home and Hospital, Findlay House, by the Daughters of Jacob Nursing Home, and Isabella Apartments by the Isabella Geriatric Center, reflected the institutional approach. Low cost housing was provided at a subsidized rental, and a "package of services," of two meals a day, social work, housekeeping and recreation services are made available at a mandatory monthly service fee. By contrast, the Kissina Apartments, sponsored by United Help-Selfhelp Community Services, represented a housing facility with services available at the option of the tenant. After considerable debate, JASA adopted a housing policy which would provide the maximum freedom of choice for elderly residents.

From the outset, JASA's housing program was designed to fulfill the following goals:

- To provide appropriately designed apartments and community facilities for the elderly at affordable rents and to maintain the elderly persons in their home for as long as possible.
- To serve the ill-housed and disadvantaged, isolated aged; to relocate the aged to a more secure environment.
- To provide supportive social services; senior citizens centers; recreational, social and cultural activities, and access to medical, psychiatric and home care services. These services would be available as the personal choice of the resident.
- To advocate for federal, state and municipal legislation to assure the aged adequate housing with supportive services (Warach, n.d.).

JASA has developed seven housing facilities, and provides management and supportive services for eight facilities, comprising ten buildings with 2,115 apartments and 2,510 elderly and handicapped tenants.

Each of the housing companies was organized as a not-for-profit housing company under Article XI of the New York State housing law, with JASA as sponsor. Between 1969 and 1986, five of the facilities with 1,118 apartments were funded by the federal Department of Housing and Urban Development, under the Section 202 direct, low interest 40-year mortgage loan program, linked to Section 8 low-income rent subsidy program. Three apartment houses were funded by the State of New York Housing Finance Agency and Urban Development Corporation, with FH236 interest subsidies, and Section 8 low income rent subsidies. All of the facilities have full or partial municipal real estate tax exemption, and are exempt from payment of sales and other business taxes.

On behalf of the National Corporation for Housing Partnerships, JASA manages Friendset House (1978), a 258-unit limited-profit housing company in Coney Island. All tenants at Friendset receive a Section 8 rent subsidy.

Over an 18-year period of development and construction, JASA housing facilities cost approximately $80 million, with $76 million in federal and state mortgage loans, and $4.3 million in philanthropic grants, contributed by three donors: the late Henry Schwartz and his Brookdale Foundation; the late S.H. and Helen R. Scheuer, and the late Evelyn and Louis A. Green. The grants were essential philanthropic equity toward paying for a portion of building site and development costs, and, particularly, additional community facilities space ordinarily not accepted for funding by state or federal housing authorities.

Elderly tenants pay affordable rents at 30 percent of their monthly income for the majority, benefiting from a Section 8 or federal rent or interest subsidy. JASA housing facilities will receive approximately $11.1 million in federal and municipal subsidies in FY 1989-90. This amounts to $5,270 per apartment per annum, or $439 per month. Direct payment by tenants will average $2,064 per annum or $172 per month. Single tenants receiving a Supplementary Security Income grant of $492 per month will pay $147.60 per month rent.

LOCATION, PLANNING AND DESIGN OF FACILITIES

Most of JASA's housing facilities and Friendset House are located in Brooklyn and Queens Shorefront areas—Coney Island, Brighton and Manhattan Beach, the Far Rockaways. One apartment house was built in Manhattan, at Cooper Square—the Bowery and 4th Street. Community facilities, the boardwalk, shopping, health services and transportation are all accessible. Three sites: Coney Island, Friendset, and the Green Residence at Cooper Square were located on Urban Development land and sold by the City of New York at a cost of $500 or less per unit. For the rest: Scheuer House of Brighton Beach was constructed on a site owned by a YM-YWHA, Scheuer House of Manhattan Beach was an old hotel, and the Brookdale Village site was acquired in the mid '60s at a very low price.

JASA's housing facilities were designed in a partnership of the architect, JASA Housing Management and JASA's social work staff. Blueprints for the apartments and community facilities incorporated advances in the "state of the art." Facilities met accessibility standards. Safety features were incorporated into the plans. Emergency communication systems connected tenants to housing management offices and resident building superintendents' apartments.

A major design emphasis was the incorporation of extensive community facilities in each building. These included a large social hall-dining room, institutional kitchen, library-conference room, arts and crafts shop, a lounge, club rooms, social work staff offices, and toilets. From the outset, state and federal funding sources, in an effort to economize, allowed no more than four to six percent of the gross square footage for community facilities. Philanthropic capital contributions paid for the additional community facilities and space. Community facilities were designed to meet the minimum space standards of the New York City Department for the Aging and the Human Resources Administration for senior citizens centers serving a minimum of 150 persons per day at lunch and other activities.

At Brookdale Village a primary care medical office is staffed by nearby St. John's Episcopal Medical Center. At Friendset House a medical office is operated by physicians affiliated with Coney Island Hospital.

These facilities made it possible to develop and operate comprehensive senior centers, tenant association activities and to provide social work counseling and care.

None of the facilities was designed to provide institutional or skilled nursing care or such services as three meals a day, medical and nursing care or physical therapy.

THE SCOPE OF MANAGEMENT AND SUPPORTIVE SERVICES IN JASA HOUSING FACILITIES

JASA's Department of Housing Development and Management has been headed by experienced housing professionals. Full-time housing managers at each facility supervise the maintenance staff and housing office operations and provide tenant services.

It was evident from the outset of JASA's housing initiative that low and moderate-income elderly residents would not have the means to pay for the supportive services. Given the scale of the JASA developments, philanthropic support would be wholly inadequate. Advocacy and planning for government funding for senior centers and services for these buildings, all located in neighborhoods densely populated by the aged, was initiated by JASA five years before completion of each project. Propitiously, increased federal, state and municipal funding of services for the aged, through Title XX of the Social Security Act (now the Social Services Block Grant), the Older Americans Act, and state and municipal programs, made it possible for JASA to secure grants to establish services in the housing facilities for both residents and other aged of the community.

Senior citizens centers at Scheuer House of Coney Island, Friendset, Scheuer House, of Manhattan Beach and Brookdale Village serve more than 1,000 elderly people a day in center activities and provide a hot lunch five days a week. Scheuer House of Brighton Beach is adjacent to the Shorefront "Y" which operates a senior center funded by the City of New York.

Caseworkers assigned by JASA to these centers and building facilities provide individual services to the elderly and the handicapped.

In 1978 the State of New York secured a Medicaid waiver to permit the provision of personal care for physically and mentally disabled persons eligible for Medicaid, or even for those somewhat above Medicaid income levels but otherwise eligible. The New York State "Expanded In-Home Service for the Elderly Program" (EISEP), and the Older Americans Act Program provide some home care for the "near poor" elderly above the Medicaid poverty level. For some homebound, a hot meal, delivered five days a week, may be secured.

During the period 1969 to 1986, once a housing facility reached 150 dwelling units, DHUD allowed funds for employment of one social worker as an expense of the housing company under the FH202 Program. This is no longer possible under present cost constraints of the federal FH202 Program.

Residents may request the assistance of JASA's social workers or be referred by JASA's housing management. Residents come to the social workers with a gamut of problems: securing a medical payment, Medicaid eligibility, even making a will. All too frequently referrals are made at a crisis when help is needed to overcome physical or mental disability, and in bereavement.

For the severely mentally impaired tenant, who is unable or refuses to accept psychiatric treatment or hospitalization, and whose family is uncooperative, the JASA social workers may request the assistance of the Protective Services Unit of the New York City department of Social Services (D.S.S.) If necessary, D.S.S. may secure an appropriate court order to require temporary hospitalization. As an alternative, psychiatric crisis intervention units of the State Department of Mental Hygiene or a voluntary organization may be called in.

Within each housing complex, JASA has assisted residents to organize tenants associations with their own elected officers and executive committees, assisted by JASA social workers. The tenants associations organize evening and weekend social, recreational and educational programs; present tenant grievances and requests to housing management, and resolve tenant problems. Volunteer "floor captains" designated for each floor, organized through the tenants associations, provide a friendly daily check on the well-being of each resident. They assist neighbors during an illness or emergency.

In essence JASA has located supportive service programs legislated for the benefit of all the aged of the neighborhood, the senior centers, social casework, the volunteers within its building facilities; but they do, indeed, serve all the elderly of the neighborhood. The close working relationship of JASA housing management and social service staff has facilitated referrals of tenants for needed services.

In New York City, funding of these services for older adults, despite reductions in federal appropriations for domestic services, has remained relatively stable. However, Federal grants for the Social Service Block Grant and the Older Americans Act have not met inflationary cost increases. Fortunately, supplementary municipal grants and increased philanthropic contributions have enabled JASA to maintain stability of services from year to year (Warach, 1986).

JASA, with a mandate to assist all of the elderly within its neighborhoods of service, is confronted with the difficult problem of priorities: Should residents of our JASA apartment houses benefit from a higher priority for services than their neighbors? Since JASA sponsors both housing *and* community-based services, the troubled and troublesome residents ask for attention from the agency's social workers, housing managers, and their neighbors—members of very effective tenants associations. And attention must be paid.

WHO ARE JASA'S RESIDENTS?

Two studies have been done on JASA's tenants. First, a "Survey of Residents of Housing Facilities Sponsored and Managed by JASA" was completed by JASA staff in 1985, and, subsequently, in 1986, "A Survey Study of Elderly Residents at Brookdale Village and the Evelyn and Louis A. Green Residence in the Rockaways" was completed by Abraham Monk, Lenard W. Kaye and Beverly Diamond, of the Brookdale Institute on Aging and Adult Human Development, Columbia University. Both confirmed the agency's appreciation of the increasing longevity of residents and the startling increase in the numbers over 75 and over 85 (Warach, 1986; Monk, Kaye, and Diamond, 1986).

HIGHLIGHTS OF THE DEMOGRAPHY OF RESIDENTS

- JASA's housing facilities had 1,814 apartments in eight buildings, 1,783 of which were occupied, reflecting a two percent vacancy rate.
- There was a total of 2,089 tenants, or 1.17 tenants per apartment.
- Of the 2,089 tenants, 1,544, 74 percent, were women; 545, or 26 percent men.
- The average age of all tenants was 77.926 years. At the oldest building, tenanted in 1967, the average age was 80.70 At the newest building, Scheuer House of Brighton Beach, the average age was 71.10.
- Some 67.4 percent of tenants, 1,407, were over 75.
- The number of tenants over 85 was 423, or 20 percent.

The average age of tenants at move-in is 72. JASA staff has concluded that, on average, residents at move-in represent a healthier, more mentally and physically stable element of the elderly population. The ability to accomplish a change of residence at age 72 requires great physical and emotional strength — a prediction of greater longevity. Applicants must be "self-maintaining."

The mental state of residents was significant as a clue to their social supports. However, for many single older residents, family could not be a source of support.

- Eleven percent of the residents, 224 persons, were single, never married.
- Twenty percent of householders, 380 persons, had had no children.
- Sixty percent of the population, or 1,261 persons, were widowed. Added to single persons, *71 percent* of the households were *one* person households.

By comparison with national data, this is a very high proportion of single person households. In 1986, only 30 percent of non-institutionalized aged lived alone.

- Of the elderly with children, 1,403 households, 79 percent, or 1,330, had children in the metropolitan area; 21 percent did not.

Thus, about one-third of the householders in tenancy (32 percent) had no adult children in the immediate area from whom to secure help or support in the event of a personal crisis.

Precise data on the physical or mental disabilities of all tenants were not available to housing management or social work staff. However, on a review of tenant records, a range of 8 to 31 percent of residents have been observed to have major physical disabilities requiring some physical aids. Monk et al. (1986) found 71.2 percent of the residents of Brookdale Village to have physical problems or illness; 22.9 percent of the tenants used home care aides to assist them with activities of daily living.

Housing managers were acutely conscious of the problems of mental disability. They reported a range of 4.3 percent to 12 percent of tenants as suffering significant mental impairment.

MAJOR PROBLEMS OF ELDERLY RESIDENTS

Chronic illness, physical impairment and mental disability have been identified as major problems of a significant number of the residents. JASA's social work staff has been fairly successful in assisting chronically ill, homebound and physically impaired residents to secure medical, home health and home attendant personal care, particularly for poor and near-poor eligible for Medicaid benefits. Social work staff has had greater difficulty in persuading some tenants with modest savings to "spend down" assets for their personal care. When impairment has become so severe as to require skilled nursing supervision, nursing home placement has occurred most often after hospitalization for a medical crisis rather than directly from home.

The mentally impaired aged have been a far greater problem for themselves, their families, fellow residents, social work and housing management staff. Bizarre and self-destructive behavior is characteristic. Self-denial of food and water leads to malnutrition, dehydration and severe illness. Unattended, turned-on faucets and stoves are dangerous. The Collier Brothers Syndrome results in filthy, insect-infested apartments. Often, refusal of relatives and the mentally impaired aged to cooperate in accepting assistance, medical care, hospitalization and relocation to an appropriate nursing home or mental hospital has made life difficult indeed for fellow tenants and staff. Relocation by legal action is very difficult to achieve in New York City.

Despite the standard tenant leases required by the State Division of Housing and Community Renewal and the federal Department or Housing and Urban Development, which provide for termination of leases for nonpayment of rent and "other good causes," enforcement in New York City is very difficult. The housing courts weigh the rights of individual tenants heavily against the rights of fellow tenants or even charitable or benign landlords. Eviction, even for just cause, for the benefit of the mentally impaired tenants, can long be delayed. Legal Aid attorneys will defend the right of the mentally impaired tenant to remain in possession of the apartment, regardless of the damage to the mentally impaired persons or their fellow tenants.

The Protective Services Unit of the Department of Social Services may secure a court order for mandatory hospitalization for a mentally impaired person where life is endangered and care is required. Ultimately, JASA's housing management may petition the Supreme Court to appoint a guardian (Committee of Person and Property) for a mentally disabled tenant. A guardian would then be legally responsible to the court to secure the most appropriate care and placement of the impaired person. This is a complex, tedious and difficult procedure. However, for some it may be the only way to secure needed care and effect the relocation of the mentally impaired tenant.

FINDING THE COMMUNITY SERVICES

At best, federally-funded housing facilities under the FH 202 Program provide for a management fee which pays for the direct costs of management. In facilities of 150 units or more, the housing facility budget may include the cost of one social worker and the utility bills and maintenance of the community facilities. In New York State-funded housing facilities, the social worker line is not an allowable cost of the housing company. Federal and state management fees are inadequate to fund supportive services. Thus, the public authority, not-for-profit agency or owner of a limited-profit housing facility must secure the money to pay for needed supportive services from other sources.

Tenants in HUD Section 202 facilities may be required to pay for mandatory meals-for programs in existence prior to 1987, but not thereafter.

The Congregate Housing Services Program (CHSP) has funded 61 projects serving 2,000 residents at a cost of $5.4 million in FY 1989. CHSP is therefore, a very limited source.

Programs in housing facilities for low-income elderly have been established by sponsors through contracts or arrangements with local departments of social services, area offices for aging and voluntary social agencies. The sources of their funding include the Older Americans Act, Title XX of the Social Services Act (Social Services Block Grant), Community

Development Block Grant, state and local tax levy funds, philanthropic funds, and modest dues, fees and contributions from older adult residents themselves.

The single cost with greatest import for frail and impaired residents is custodial personal care at home. Such costs can be catastrophic to the elderly retiree on fixed income with modest assets. Where states have requested Medicaid waivers, as in New York, these services can be secured for the poorest impaired aged.

Sponsors of housing facilities may enlist the cooperation of government and voluntary agencies as partners in the effort to provide support services for the elderly residents. It is to be hoped that the management plans submitted to federal and state housing offices prior to approval of the project for mortgage financing include a sound plan for provision of services. With determined effort by the professional management of housing facilities a significant program can be developed and maintained.

SECURING THE RESOURCES
TO DEVELOP ADDITIONAL FACILITIES
FOR LOW AND MODERATE INCOME ELDERLY

JASA has more than 8,000 applications for its housing facilities. With a rate of turnover of seven percent annually, there are about 140 apartment vacancies a year. This is not surprising. There are tens of thousands of elderly applicants for the 48,000 apartments at similar facilities sponsored by other voluntary agencies, limited-profit sponsors and the Housing Authority in New York City.

The Housing and Community Development Act of 1987 authorized 12,000 Section FH 202 units for FY 1988 and FY 1989. However, economies required by the Gramm-Rudman Act reduced the allocation in FY 1988 to 10,990 units, with the direct loan limitation at $565.8 million (Special Committee on Aging, 1987). Twenty-five percent of this loan authority money must be used for the handicapped. The President's budget for FY 1989 proposed a reduction of 50.9 percent, with loan authorization at $286.6 million. For FY 89 Congress appropriated $40 million to support 9,500 (Select Committee on Aging, 1988) elderly and 2,000 units for the handicapped (Older Americans Report, 1988). For all of New York State, funding levels in FY 1987-88 for FH202 programs amounted to a total of 1,462 units with an allocation of $73,482,700. New York City and its suburban counties received 1,070 units at $58,575,000 (The Daily News, 1987).

During the last three years the acquisition of a building site zoned to provide the right to construct 100 or more units in middle class areas of the New York metropolitan area has become very difficult. Costs exceed $120 a square foot, which can mean a price of $2.4 million for a 20,000 square foot site to construct 150 units. The maximum HUD allowable cost for FH 202 projects in recent years has been $500 per dwelling unit or $75,000 for the site. The only sites available are owned by the City in urban redevelopment areas. This option for site acquisition has been followed by some non-profit developers. Churches, synagogues or other institutions with surplus land and imbued with a concern for the elderly have sold or contributed sites for housing development, often becoming sponsors.

Given the soaring costs of housing construction in the New York area, with development costs for high-rise construction exceeding $150 per square foot, and the continued reduction in government mortgage loan and rent subsidy programs, the immediate outlook for production of new housing for the elderly is grim.

THE DEVELOPMENT AND MANAGEMENT OF HOUSING AND RETIREE COMMUNITIES FOR MIDDLE AND UPPER INCOME ELDERLY

The private sector has taken the initiative in development, sale and management of housing facilities which range from low cost boarding houses for the elderly to expensive retirement life care communities. These communities, originally located in the sun belt states, are now evident in the outer urban ring of metropolitan areas in Illinois, Michigan, New Jersey, New York and Pennsylvania. They offer independent housing and a range of services including security guards, building maintenance, social and recreational activities and facilities, and transportation. Fifteen years ago, in 1976, there were an estimated 2,363 retirement communities in the United States, housing almost one million residents (Marcus et al., 1983).

In the life care communities a continuum of health, personal care and nursing services may be offered. There are an estimated 300 to 600 life care communities; 300 serve 90,000 persons (Special Committee on Aging, 1987). Most life care communities are operated by private, non-profit agencies and religious organizations. There is interest in the business sector in developing and operating such facilities. While most life care communities, by all reports, have been managed effectively, there have been some grave defaults. The State of New York does not yet permit establishment of life care communities which require a non-recoverable investment of capital to purchase admission to a life care facility. Given the uncertainties of inflationary cost increases, particularly health and supportive services with a high personal service component, and the probability of a continued increase in longevity, life care communities cannot provide absolute assurance for coverage of all service and long-term care costs.

The greatest number of housing units are being produced as retirement facilities in which real estate costs, maintenance and services are uncoupled sources, with housing developers taking the lead. In New York's Suffolk County, several thousand units have been constructed in retirement communities at costs of $250,000 to $350,000 per house. Maintenance services and amenities are attractive offerings, but, by all reports, sales are going slowly.

JASA and other non-profit agencies involved in housing for the elderly have considered development of housing for middle-income elderly. The great business risks for the developer weigh heavily against such direct participation. JASA has recently explored a cooperative venture with a real estate developer.

For the time being, the building industry is producing sufficient housing units to satisfy the market demands of middle class elderly for retirement residences. However, the recent increases in mortgage interest rates and slow sales will discourage new housing production.

ARE THERE OTHER INITIATIVES
IN HOUSING PROGRAMS FOR THE ELDERLY?

In recent years, with the curtailment of new housing development, greater attention has been paid to alternative opportunities to assist the elderly to retain their own homes and apartments, and to assure their continued occupancy, adequate maintenance, and installation of health, safety and security devices. It has long been recognized that most elderly will, after all, grow older in their long time homes and will *not* relocate. There is great comfort in familiar surroundings, amongst friends and neighbors, even in changed neighborhoods (Myers, 1983).

During the past 22 years, JASA has assisted thousands of elderly persons to leave disintegrating, crime-ridden areas and to relocate to its own housing facilities and other new large scale developments, such as Rochdale Village, Starrett City and Co-op City. However, many elderly stayed on in their old neighborhoods, secure in a rent controlled apartment. In more recent years some of these neighborhoods have been gentrified and other problems have arisen from the effort of landlords to displace elderly tenants from low-rent apartments. This has been observed especially in areas with three-family homes not protected by rent control.

JASA social workers have assisted elderly tenants by persuading landlords to repair apartments by providing cash grants to poor aged to install grab bars in bathrooms, security locks for doors, and by obtaining the City funded benefit of "Senior Citizen Rent Increase Exceptions." House owners have been assisted to secure "circuit breaker" tax relief, or "Real Estate Tax Exemption for Senior Citizens," or "Home Energy Assistance Grants."

In 1987, JASA initiated a home sharing program in Queens, funded by the city and state. This modest experiment, staffed by one social worker, has succeeded in relocating elderly persons in homes and apartments. Given the availability of unused bedrooms amongst elderly "empty nesters," home sharing is a constructive option which should be pursued.

Other initiatives in the State of New York, such as the "Enriched Housing Program," funded by state Supplementary Security benefits, provide domiciliary care for impaired or frail poor elderly in small apartment residences. A modest number of congregate housing facilities has been developed within the state.

With the shortage of affordable housing in New York City and its suburbs, there has been an observed increase in development of legal and illegal accessory apartments, particularly in areas zoned for one-family homes. Elderly families have provided accessory apartments for younger families, or moved into such apartments themselves. There has been an increasing incidence of community conflict in the effort to secure zoning amendments.

Undoubtedly, public and voluntary agencies, and the private sector, need to accord a far greater priority to efforts to assist the elderly to enjoy continued occupancy of their homes and adaptation for better living to advanced old age (New York State Division of Housing and Community Renewal, 1986; Pollack and Malakoff, 1986).

CLOSING THE GAP:
PUBLIC POLICY AND LEGISLATION
FOR A BETTER OLD AGE

The facts about the aging-in of older Americans are plainly before us. The added years of life are an opportunity and a great benefit, but have created new problems. Many elderly are still assisted by family and friends, but millions have no spouse, no children and are far removed from family. They need personal care at home. Though we have made progress, millions of older Americans are still ill-housed. Poor and middle-income elderly cannot pay market rents for better housing even it is available. Since most older people will, within the next decade, live out their allotted time in their own homes, ways and means must be found to improve houses and apartments, and to provide support services in place.

No single program will satisfy the enormous range of age related housing problems, or "Aging In Place." Nor will any single group of providers satisfy such a service need. Government, the voluntary and private sectors and the business economy must, and will, participate in this national effort. But, clearly, the problems of the elderly are national in scope and will require the remedy of federal and state legislation. The leadership of the housing for the elderly movement should continue its advocacy for federal and state legislation to provide for the following major programs:

- A national long-term care insurance program under Medicare, with universal coverage for the poor and disabled, to meet the costs of community-based social, medical and rehabilitative care, home care, adult day centers, or nursing home care.
- Restoration of the Section 202 direct loan program to fund production of 40,000 housing units annually.
- An amended Section 8 Program to extend rental subsidies beyond 20 years. Expiration of these contracts, without alternative funding of rent subsidies, threatens elderly residents with eviction because of their inability to pay market rents or the wholesale foreclosure of housing projects.
- Amend legislation to avert prepayment of federal mortgages and removal of subsidized housing units from use by low-income elderly.
- Increase federal appropriations for the Congregate Care Program (CHSP) to the authorized level of $10 million per annum in fiscal 1989 and to higher levels thereafter.
- Increase authorized management fees by one or more percent in federal and state funded housing for the elderly facilities, to fund one social worker per 100 dwelling units. All housing management plans should be amended to include a plan for development and provision of supportive services for frail and impaired residents.
- Provide increased federal appropriations for flexible subsidies to restore and rehabilitate all housing for the elderly facilities and public housing to acceptable standards of physical condition.
- Restore tax incentives for the building industry to develop additional housing units for poor and moderate income elderly.

- Provide additional, earmarked funding of the Older Americans Act to strengthen the provision of existing housing by funding programs for home sharing, moderate repairs, accessibility, and installation of safety services.
- Federal and state legislation is needed to facilitate home equity conversion programs.
- State governments should be urged to establish or strengthen state mortgage loan programs for production of additional housing units for low and moderate-income elderly (Gozonsky, 1988; National Council on the Aging, 1988; National Housing Conference, 1988a, 1988b).

There has been great progress in the development and management of assisted housing and services enjoyed by millions of older Americans. These programs came to pass because of the advocacy of concerned citizens and professionals in the housing movement, and a responsive government. With continued advocacy, the housing for the elderly program can once again be funded at or near adequate levels to meet the needs of our ever increasing aged population.

REFERENCES

Gozonsky, M. "On-Again/Off-Again Housing Bill . . . On-Again." (Spring 1988). *BNAI BRITH Housing for Seniors.* Washington, DC: Bnai Brith Housing Committee, Bnai Brith International.

Marcus, R.W., Feldt, G., Pastalan, L.A., Hunt, M.E.., and Vakalo, K.L. (1983). "Retirement Communities: Present and Future." In Urban Land Institute, *Housing for a Maturing Population*, Washington, DC. Urban Land Institute.

Monk, A., Kaye, L.W., and Diamond, B. (1986). *A Survey Study of Elderly Residents at Brookdale Village and the Evelyn and Louis A. Green Residence.* Sponsored and managed by the Jewish Association for Services for the Aged. New York, NY: Brookdale Institute on Aging and Adult Human Development, Columbia University.

Myers, P. (1983). "Gentrification of the Elderly: Aging in Place." In the Urban Land Institute, *Housing for a Maturing Population*. Washington, DC: Urban Land Institute.

National Council on the Aging. (1988). "Public Policy Agenda 1988-1989 of the National Council on the Aging, Inc." *Perspectives on Aging*, XVII (2).

National Housing Conference. (1988a). "NHC Reports from Washington." *Conference Review*, 57 (3). Washington, DC: National Housing Conference.

National Housing Conference. (1988b). "NHC Reports from Washington." *Conference Review*, 57 (4). Washington, DC: National Housing Conference.

New York State Division of Housing and Community Renewal. (1986). *SHOP Shared Housing Option Program, Progress and Prospects*. Albany, NY: New York State Division of Housing and Urban Renewal.

Older Americans Report. (May 27, 1988). 12 (22), 217. Silver Springs, MD: Business Publishers, Inc.

Pollack, P.B. and Malakoff, L.Z . (1986). *Housing Options for Older New Yorkers: A Source Book*. Ithaca and Albany, NY: Cornell Cooperative Extension and the New York State Office for the Aging.

Select Committee on Aging, U.S. House of Representatives. (1988). "Section 202 Housing Budget Crisis: A Report by the Chairman." Publication No. 100-682. Washington, DC: U.S. Government Printing Office.

Special Committee on Aging, U.S. Senate. (1987). *Developments in Aging: 1987, Volume I*. Washington, DC: U.S. Government Printing Office.

The Daily News. (October 1, 1987). New York, NY: the Daily News.

Warach, B. (1986). "Supportive Services in Housing for the Elderly: Emerging Needs and Problems." *Journal of Jewish Communal Service*, 62 (4), 299-306.

Warach, B. (n.d.). "Housing an Aging Society Emerging Issues," Conference on Housing an Aging Society. Sponsored by the U.S. Department of Housing and Urban Development and the Mortgage Bankers Association of New Jersey, Monmouth College, New Jersey.

An Offer They Could Not Refuse:
Housing for the Elderly

Thomas J. Fairchild
David P. Higgins
W. Edward Folts

The growth of the older population in America has attracted the attention of a number of real estate developers, hotel chains, and other proprietary companies and has created what Minkler (1989, p. 19) calls the "geriatric social industrial complex." The rush to develop service model retirement communities has caused a shock wave in the $4-billion-plus retirement housing industry (Fairchild, 1987). Interest in the senior market and in retirement housing specifically has grown dramatically during the past decade. In recent years, much attention has been devoted to aging Americans in the popular press and in various trade publications targeted at real estate developers and companies in the hospitality business (Knowlton, 1988). Non-profit organizations that have long dominated the retirement community market now find that they must compete with proprietary companies. This paper, however, will not discuss the impact of proprietary companies that were involved in providing health care services

Thomas J. Fairchild, PhD, is Director and Associate Professor at the Center for Studies in Aging, University of North Texas. His current focus is in the area of retirement housing and long-term care, and he has done research in the area of staffing issues in retirement housing and health care. Dr. Fairchild has worked with a variety of sponsors, developers, and architects in the area of retirement housing. David P. Higgins, PhD, is Associate Professor of Finance and Director of the Corporate Finance MBA Program at the University of Dallas, Irving, TX. His interest is in financing of long-term care, from both provider and user perspectives. He has been a member of the faculty at Arizona State University and the University of Wisconsin. W. Edward Folts, PhD, is Associate Professor in the Department of Sociology and Social Work, Appalachian State University, Boone, NC. His current focus is in the area of nontraditional alternative housing arrangements. Dr. Folts received his PhD from the University of Florida.

and housing for seniors prior to the late 1970s. Because of their involvement, most of these companies have created an established niche for themselves in the nursing home and/or housing market. What this experience reflects is an identification with a set of products and services that constitute the core business of most of these companies or, in a few cases, diversification that is consistent with their business objectives.

Furthermore, although a number of investor-owned companies have entered the retirement housing marketplace in the past 10 years, this phenomenon can perhaps best be characterized by the activity of companies that represent builders/developers and the hospitality industry. The companies that are representative of these two types of businesses clearly have had the greatest impact on the retirement housing industry over the past decade. By their presence in the market they have started to redefine retirement housing, and their impact will likely last for many years to come. Therefore, the discussion that follows will focus on the activities of these companies, review the reasons why for-profit companies have entered the retirement housing field, and examine the type of housing products that they have built for Americans 65 years of age and older over the past decade. Finally, this paper will explore what the future might hold for investor-owned companies in the retirement housing field.

THE DECADE OF THE 1980s —
THE REASONS

In order to have a full appreciation of the type of housing products that builders/developers and companies in the hotel business have constructed, mostly since the mid-1980s, it is important to understand the reasons why many of these companies entered the senior housing market during the last 10 years. As the decade of the 1990s begins, "aging is in." A recent article in *Fortune* (Fischer, 1990, p. 108) states, "Certainly marketers must be aware of overlooking a remarkably vigorous, diverse, and well-to-do group — consumers over 50." This same article goes on to suggest that "the market for care of the elderly will grow apace" (p. 109).

The discovery of the "gero-market" occurred for most of the business world approximately a decade ago, when a few national business publications and the popular press started to write about the "Graying of America." The dynamics of this population change in the first part of the 1980s were given increased priority in the trade publications read by developers, bankers, marketers, and executives in the hospitality industry. Many of these same business persons were noting that "people aged 55 and over control about one-third of the discretionary income in the United States and spend 30% in the marketplace" (Kaplan & Longino, 1989, p. 13). In fact, because of the increased exposure of the private sector to the march of the Baby Boomers toward Golden Pond, the Graying of America was hardly considered a new phenomenon by the mid-1980s (Fairchild & Folts, 1989a).

The search for "gold in them gray hills" had begun in earnest by the time two other economic "drivers of change" started to have a significant impact on the U.S. economy. The dramatic growth of the elderly population tipped the development scales for a number of for-profit companies, who entered the retirement housing market with a rush. It was during the same period of the decade that the demand for commercial real estate began to decline. The portfolio of many developers started to bulge with properties that had too few tenants and too large a debt service. Many properties were finished but never occupied. Tax reform, which had a direct and negative impact on real estate tax incentives, was a major blow to the real estate industry. Although there was considerable debate about the reasons for this predicament in real estate circles, most analysts were pessimistic about the future of commercial real estate. Most types of commercial real estate had been overbuilt in many areas of the United States, and as a result only companies with very "deep pockets" could expect to survive the years ahead. A number of real estate development companies (e.g., Southmark) with years of experience in the marketplace found themselves faced with default and bankruptcy. As the shakeout started, developers were looking for any way they could to survive. The lifeline for some of them appeared to be housing built for people 65 years of age and older. Those empty office buildings started to look more like retirement housing, and the tracts of land purchased for office parks looked perfect for retirement communities.

A second "driver of change" that altered the face of the retirement housing industry was the overcapacity that was starting to become evident to executives in the lodging industry. As early as 1979, hotel growth was outpacing demand. "To remain profitable, hotels generally need to fill 70 percent of their rooms—a level they haven't reached since 1979" (Gutis, 1990, p. 8). In order to respond to this looming crisis, the hotel industry tried developing new products to fill market niches like all-suite hotels and started catering more and more to business travelers by offering services like FAX machines and creating business centers within the hotel (Winans, 1989). Nevertheless, the decline continued to worsen, and by the mid-1980s analysts were predicting that the situation would not improve until the middle of the 1990s. The shakeout that characterized the real estate industry in the late 1970s to mid-1980s was now predicted to occur in the hotel market by the late 1980s and early 1990s (Chakravarty, 1987; Gutis, 1990). The strategy that a number of companies chose to pursue in order to deal with this problem was to follow the demographic age wave and start to develop housing products that would care for the shelter needs of the elderly. Perhaps this approach is best characterized by an executive vice-president from a leading company in the hospitality industry, who said, "In all other businesses we have to sell people every day to get them to come in. We think it's great to have the same person to take care of every day" (Chakravarty, 1987, p. 113).

What distinguishes the companies that entered the senior housing market beginning in the late 1970s from those that had been involved prior to that time was that they were attempting to capitalize on the senior boom by developing a group of housing products and services for a market in which they had little, if any, prior experience. Initially, this effort at diversification was marked more by the need to remain financially sound than by a desire to learn about aging and then apply this knowledge to address the housing needs of people over the age of 65. Companies in the hotel business felt that meeting the housing needs of seniors was a very natural extension of their current business (Amparano, 1988; Carnevale, 1989; Peterson, 1989). Retirement housing for companies in the hotel field was seen as "a line extension — another brand in the family" (Gutis, 1990, p. 8).

Developers, on the other hand, did not have this edge. They were not accustomed to taking care of people. Where their experience rested was on the "bricks and mortar" side of the business. They knew how to build and, in some cases, manage buildings. Armed with this experience and the developer's propensity to be willing to "walk on thin ice," they felt more or less prepared to enter the housing market for seniors.

THE PRODUCT

Working from their strengths and the "blind optimism" that resulted from "early successes with congregate-care operations in the late 1970s" (Celis, 1988, p. 19), proprietary companies started to build various types of retirement housing. Many of the original facilities were conceived as large-scale luxury communities targeted at healthy, upper-income couples in the 65 to 74 age range.

The facilities that were being built in the early 1980s — often referred to as congregate care housing — offered dining, housekeeping, and transportation services. In addition, they provided the residents with a variety of entertainment and activity programs. Generally, these communities made no provision for health care and provided little assistance with daily activities such as bathing and dressing. They were essentially apartments that offered a select number of necessary services. Most of the properties that were developed used a rental approach rather than charging an entrance fee. This was a very significant development because, with the exception of projects sponsored by the U.S. Department of Housing and Urban Development, very few rental options had been available to elderly people with middle to upper incomes. Most of these new facilities provided little in the way of health care (e.g., nursing home services) and focused on the independent living end of the housing continuum. The projects built in the early 1980s reflected a view of the elderly as a couple between the ages of 65 and 74 who required few health or social services. These early facilities were primarily the outcome of the attitude of builders and developers who thought they could be successful if they added a restaurant to apartment units.

The obvious relationship between independent living, assisted living, and nursing homes had not yet penetrated the mind-set or business plans of these new players in the retirement housing field. As a result of this approach, the new buzzword became "aging in place" (Fairchild & Folts, 1989b, p. 10). The challenge for the operators of new projects was how to provide additional health and social services to residents whose frailty level was increasing faster then they had anticipated in a building that was not designed for such levels of support.

The experience of these developers did not go completely unnoticed by some of the newcomers who were about to enter the retirement housing market. Some observers of the industry noted that, "during the past several years, the most important trend in the retirement center industry has been its growing sensitivity to various segments of the elderly population" (Graham, 1987a, p. 52). The vocabulary of for-profits began to expand to include words like "widow," "social services," "activities of daily living," "assisted living," "congregate care," "nursing homes," and "continuum of care." The importance of providing the resident with assistance in activities of daily living and access to health care services started to be recognized by proprietary companies.

The realization that long-term care/retirement housing "is more than breaking ground and building properties" (Taninecz, 1988, p. 115) was perhaps first accepted by some of the hospitality companies that were starting to develop retirement housing (Amparano, 1988; Ricklefs, 1988; Winans, 1989). A number of executives from some of these firms came to understand that "the hotel adage, 'heads in beds,' just doesn't cut it when you're talking about taking this country's elderly into the sunset" (Taninecz, 1988, p. 115). The move in this direction was facilitated by the fact that for-profits were able to develop numerous methods "to eliminate or reduce the amount of taxes they [paid] on the initial fees" (Barody & Buckles, 1989, p. 13) and therefore began using the entrance fee approach to finance continuing care retirement communities (CCRCs). For some projects, these fees were up to 90% refundable and might range from approximately $125,000 to $200,000 with monthly fees from $1,120 to $2,225 (Taninecz, 1988). This change was extremely significant because, for the first time, it enabled for-profits to develop facilities that offered a continuum of care and used an entrance fee structure.

The development of rental retirement projects offering different levels of care also started to become more popular (Seip, 1987), and the importance of slicing the market into groups that differed by age and need began to gain acceptance by for-profit companies. While some newcomers moved ahead with facilities offering housing only for independent seniors, new products started to be built that included a "full continuum of care — from independent living to assisted living and skilled nursing" (Seip, 1987, p. 49). Such facilities were better designed to meet the social and health care needs of the prospective resident who, more often than not, was a widow in her late 70s (Clunn, Kopp, & Lasman, 1987).

Many of these projects used a rental approach rather than an entrance fee structure. Therefore, by the mid-1980s, the market included CCRCs that were operated by proprietary companies and were using either an entrance fee or monthly rental fee structure. Because of the levels of housing and health care that the new facilities included, they were able to compete directly with more established non-profit facilities. Although the new communities did not immediately threaten non-profit operators, the non-profits were clearly interested in how these retirement centers would be accepted by the elderly. As an executive of a leading non-profit multi-facility company said, "much of what they do could set a new and higher set of expectations for the elderly" (Graham, 1987b, p. 116).

Acceptance of the natural link between independent living, assisted living, and nursing care, however, was not universal. Even though more for-profit facilities were being built during the mid-1980s that offered a range of housing and service options, projects without a continuum of care were still being planned and developed. The congregate care retirement model of the late 1970s and early 1980s was still seen as an acceptable housing product even though the market for this type of housing was "smaller than anticipated and some developers . . . misjudged the type of facilities that would draw well-off retirees" (Celis, 1988, p. 19). A related problem that pushed some new players to build other, more supportive products was the fact that over three-quarters of the housing that had been built since the early 1980s was designed for affluent elderly, who made up only about 20% of the elderly population (Celis, 1988).

THE FUTURE

By the time the 1980s were drawing to a close, for-profits had clearly set the stage on which they would play for the foreseeable future. In the waning years of the decade they tried a few new twists like combining the benefits of condominium ownership with on-campus health facilities (Adams & Benderoff, 1988; Dannenfeldt, 1989). These efforts, however, did very little to change the direction that they had set in the early to mid-1980s.

The state of the retirement housing industry from the viewpoint of the proprietary sector is perhaps best summed up in a recent editorial by Gamzon (1990) in *Multi-Housing News* titled "The Next 'Up-Cycle' and Beyond." Gamzon argues that the experience of participants in the senior housing industry over the past few years has resulted in a situation in which those participants have "struggled to understand the unique nature of the heterogeneous seniors markets" (p. 60). Most, but not all, newcomers had realized by the late 1980s that congregate facilities without health services will not meet the needs of many seniors and therefore will not be financially viable. They further realized that, because they did not "listen to gerontologists and health care planners" (Gamzon, 1990, p. 60), they failed to recognize the design and operational impact of aging in place. They entered the senior housing market with the expressed goal "to create a structure to provide leadership to an industry that's been fraught with inconsistency" (Taninecz, 1988, p. 114). Their experience was a humbling one. Many of the original developers of congregate-care products have retreated to their original markets. Many areas of the country are overbuilt with a product that very few elderly need or want. The result of this continued overbuilding has been more lender losses, more troubled properties, and an increase in state regulations governing the contract content of retirement communities (Netting & Wilson, 1987).

The market is undergoing a shakeout and, hence, consolidation. The goal of for-profit developers and companies from the hospitality industry to give the retirement housing field leadership and direction has yet to be achieved. In fact, rather than adding greater clarity to the industry, their involvement has resulted in more confusion.

Perhaps the single biggest question that remains is whether for-profit companies have come to understand that success in the retirement housing business is dependent upon their ability to blend "care and cash" concerns. Projects built in the next decade must offer "a practical 'continuum of care' that recognizes aging-in-place as a natural component in the aging process" (Fairchild, Dunkelman, & Folts, 1989, p. 12). The companies that have been successful over the past 30 years have realized that providing housing to the elderly is an "inside-out business." They have accepted the fact that the focus of management must begin inside the facility with the individual, not outside with marketing, bricks, and mortar. Providing retirement housing is a service business, and it requires a management team that understands that the most important word in the phrase "continuing care retirement community" is "care." This understanding necessitates an understanding of health care, an area where few for-profit newcomers have desired to tread.

In the area of retirement housing, the 1990s, like the 1980s, will be full of unknowns and surprises, but some things are certain. The pace of change in retirement housing will be faster, and competition will intensify. Yet, as much as we talk about change in the retirement housing industry during the next decade, it would be helpful to keep in mind the words of noted futurist Daniel Bell (1967, cited in Fairchild & Burton, 1982, p. 84): "The world of the year 2000 has already arrived, for in the decisions we make now, in the way we design our environment and thus sketch the lines of constraints, the future is committed."

REFERENCES

Adams, E., & Benderoff, E. L. (1988, July). Services for seniors. *Professional Builder.* pp. 72-83.

Amparano, J. (1988, February 11). Marriott sees green in catering to a graying nation. *The Wall Street Journal,* p. 11.

Barody, M., & Buckles, W. G., Jr. (1989). Southern management says CCRCs here to stay. *Provider, 15*(9), 13-15.

Carnevale, M. (1989, July 21). Marriott to build 150 retirement sites at cost of $1 billion in next 5 years. *The Wall Street Journal,* p. 5.

Celis, W., III. (1988, August 3). "Congregate care" housing is overbuilt in some areas. *The Wall Street Journal,* p. 19.

Chakravarty, S. N. (1987, November 30). Sails reefed. *Forbes,* pp. 110, 111, 113.

Clunn, B. A., Kopp, W. C., & Lasman, G. A. (1987, March/April). Retirement centers: Where housing meets healthcare. *Healthcare Executive,* pp. 44-48.

Dannenfeldt, D. (1989). Hospitals wary about retirement ventures. *Modern Healthcare, 19* (42), 44, 46.

Fairchild, T. J. (1987). The future of the retirement housing industry: Bust or boom? *Contemporary Long-Term Care, 10*(6), 72, 74-75, 77.

Fairchild, T. J., & Burton, B. S. (1982). Aging in the year 2000. In N. S. Ernst & H. Glazer-Waldman (Eds.), *The aging patient: A sourcebook for the allied health professional* (pp. 84-97). Chicago: Year Book Publications.

Fairchild, T. J., Dunkelman, D., & Folts, W. E. (1989). The forces of change: Elderly housing in the 21st century. *Retirement Housing Report, 4*(1), 11-12.

Fairchild, T. J., & Folts, W. E. (1989a). Elder housing in the 1990s: Problem or opportunity? *The Southwestern. 5*(2), 10-18.

Fairchild, T. J., & Folts, W. E. (1989b). Managing the impact of aging residents and facilities. In *Retirement housing industry 1988* (pp. 10-11). Philadelphia: Laventhol & Horwath.

Fischer, A. B. (1990, January, 29). What consumers want in the 1990s. *Fortune.* pp. 108-112.

Gamzon, M. (1990, January). The next "up-cycle" and beyond. *Multi-Housing News,* p. 60.

Graham, J. (1987a). Demand should foster rapid growth in retirement center industry experts. *Modern Healthcare. 17*(9), 52, 58.

Graham, J. (1987b). Retirement centers increase in numbers in effort to accommodate affluent elderly. *Modern Healthcare. 17*(12), 112, 114, 116.

Gutis, P. S. (1990, April 8). After a decade of growth, far too much room at the inn. *The New York Times,* p. 8.

Kaplan, K. M., & Longino, C. (1989, May/June). Gray in gold: A public-private conundrum. *The Spectrum.* pp. 13-15.

Knowlton, C. (1988, September 26). Consumers: A tougher sell. *Fortune,* pp. 65, 66, 70, 74.

Minkler, M. (1989). Gold in gray: Reflections on business' discovery of the elderly market. *The Gerontologist, 29,* 17-23.

Netting, F. E., & Wilson, C. C. (1987). Current legislation concerning life care and continuing care contracts. *The Gerontologist, 27,* 645-651.

Peterson, I. (1989, July 30). Hotel chains plunge into life-care field. *The New York Times.* pp. 1, 11.

Ricklefs, R. (1988, November 25). Communities for aged offer "total security," but with trade-offs. *The Wall Street Journal,* p. 1.

Seip, D. E. (1987). 1987: An insider's perspective on the retirement industry. *Contemporary Long-Term Care, 10*(12), 48-49.

Taninecz, G. (1988, April 18). Hotel companies test market for long-term care of elderly. *Hotel and Motel Management,* pp. 1, 114-116.

Winans, C. (1989, November 28). Lodging chains sour on all-suite hotel. *The Wall Street Journal,* pp. 1, 14.

IV. FUTURE PERSPECTIVES

A Future Agenda
for Congregate Housing Research

M. Powell Lawton

This chapter will use the contributions to this volume as a starting point for some thoughts about research needs in congregate housing. Although this chapter is not the place for it, if one set about to review past research specific to congregate housing, not a great deal of space would be required. The fact is that while much research has been concerned with housing for older people, relatively little has focused on the attributes that define congregate housing as a genre. In an attempt to encourage such a focus for the future, this chapter will define researchable problems that are generic specifically to congregate housing more than to other types of housing, or research issues that help articulate the attributes of congregate housing by comparing it to other types of housing.

SEVEN CATEGORIES OF RESEARCH NEEDS

Because congregate housing has stimulated relatively little research to date, there is a continuing need for descriptive research of two kinds. The

M. Powell Lawton, PhD, is a clinical psychologist and Director of the Polisher Research Institute of the Philadelphia Geriatric Center. His research has emphasized the environmental psychology of later life, assessment of the elderly, and mental health issues.

first is purely demographic in terms of a data base that tracks the basic characteristics of all congregate housing. The second type of descriptive research is cost-oriented research. Three other categories constitute what might be called "process" research, research designed to tell us what goes on in congregate housing. One type of process concerns the physical design features that support or impede achieving the goals of congregate housing. Second is research on management of congregate housing. The last process feature is the organization and delivery of services in the housing. Another of the research categories concerns the ultimate outcomes associated with living in congregate housing, and the quality of life and health that accrues to residents of this type of housing. Finally are policy issues that may be elucidated by the analysis of large-scale data sets. Each of these seven categories of research need will be discussed in turn.

DESCRIPTIVE MONITORING
OF CONGREGATE HOUSING

It is very significant that none of the papers in this collection is based on a representative or a large-sized sample of congregate housing sites. Data from old surveys (Office of Policy Development and Research, 1979; Malozemoff, Anderson, & Rosenbaum, 1978) are still being cited as the major multi-site studies, or special-purpose surveys such as the Congregate Housing Services Program (CHSP, Sherwood et al., 1985) or the residential care survey (Mor, Sherwood, & Gutkin, 1986). Major impediments to performing new research of this kind are the lack, first, of a consensual definition of congregate housing and, second, of a register from which a researcher may draw a sample of congregate housing for study. A number of issues relating to the need for archival information in housing for the older person have been discussed elsewhere (Lawton, 1990).

Thus a first research need is a data base from which basic descriptive information regarding congregate housing may be obtained. The American Association of Homes for the Aged (Continuing Care Retirement Communities, 1987; 1989) has the best start on this endeavor in its biennial survey of Continuing Care Retirement Communities (CCRC). This data base contains a great deal of useful information on the structural, organizational, financial, and service-delivery aspects of retirement communities. Although the survey is not limited to AAHA members, it does not include proprietary communities nor any of the varieties of congregate housing without the guarantee (either in prepaid or pay-as-you-go form) of life care from independent housing to nursing care. The commercially-published *National Directory of Retirement Facilities* (1988) may well constitute the most complete listing of congregate housing now available because of its effort to track new communities as they are added to the total pool, through a variety of sources. This listing also has limitations in representativeness; its entries are of as yet unknown reliability as sources of research-usable data on operating and service-related characteristics. This publication is not a good guide to the presence of congregate services because some facilities provide extensive listings while other facilities provide none.

Should support become available to alter this data base or create a new data base for research purposes, some issues requiring attention would be:

- Another definition of congregate housing would need to be provided.
- Inclusionary criteria are needed to make certain that the major types of congregate housing appear: CCRCs, proprietary congregate residences, free-standing congregate housing under both public and nonprofit sponsorship.
- Exclusionary criteria that would eliminate quasi-institutions such as board and care, domiciliary care, and small-group residences designed for full support of Alzheimer patients and other special groups, are also needed.
- Decisions regarding whether to include or exclude "residential care" settings where no kitchen facilities exist; congregate services programs targeted to only a segment of the total population, as in CHSP; and many forms of "alternative housing."
- An approach is required to provide guidance to the user regarding how to deal with the biases of nonresponse or incomplete enumeration of the universe. Even the most favorable situation, the AAHA data base, manages to obtain only about a 50% response rate from eligible CCRCs.
- Decisions about the scope of information feasible to include on a data base. The AAHA experience is helpful here, in that only the most basic data are requested, yet responding institutions agree that even this amount of data retrieval puts a substantial burden on them.

Basic Descriptive Characteristics

A first-level minimum data set should include factual information on sponsorship, geographic and urban-rural location, number of units by unit size and residents, age of community, building types, fee structure (as indicated, entrance fee, range of monthly rent or maintenance fee by unit type, purchase cost, unbundled rent), contractual type, presence of other levels of housing or care, licensure status, and availability of a short list of supportive services, with costs.

A second, more detailed level would add information about staff and resident characteristics. These items require new work to count and aggregate by types and are frequently the basis for a facility's choosing not to respond to a questionnaire.

The most complex level of data are items best left to survey research methods where face-to-face or possibly telephone interviews can be conducted. Much of the most useful information on costs, administrative practices, programs, physical amenities available, resident movement, and many types of changes over time fall into this category.

Cost-Oriented Research

Heumann's (this issue) chapter is the best possible illustration of the complexities of cost-oriented research. Heumann is totally correct in pointing out the types of oversimplification that have made many previous attempts to test the cost-effectiveness of congregate housing suspect. There may even have been a negative political effect resulting from the too-easy conclusions about the cost superiority of congregate housing that early research unconcerned with equating risk factors produced.

Necessary cost-oriented research goes far beyond comparing congregate housing and institutional care, however. A great deal of the data on long term financial health of CCRCs is in the hands of proprietary entities at this point. With consulting services to sell, it is understandable why the consultant corporations have not placed these specific data in the public domain. AAHA is building up its own bank of such data, however, which is projected to be made accessible to both operational entities and researchers.

There are many specific issues regarding costs that require new research. Examples include exploring the most cost-beneficial ways of offering meal services in congregate housing. Sponsors are in great need of means of projecting the net costs of different options for meal services ranging from the totally bundled monthly fee that includes all meals for all residents to the other end of the continuum where taking meals is totally elective. Another need is to provide guidelines from the experiences of various housing types regarding the tradeoffs associated with having all services organized and directed by local management as compared to being contracted out to specialist providers.

In both of these examples as well as in other cost-oriented research, the problems are complicated by psychological costs and benefits associated with different cost-related alternatives. Having a choice about whether to buy housing-provided meals has often been suggested as having a major positive psychological impact. Research is needed, however, to tell us whether a time comes in people's physical competence, or whether some people's personality needs are such that having this type of decision-making and control are of low importance.

The ideally most-productive type of large-scale survey of congregate housing should begin by attempting to improve the current master lists of facilities to form a sampling frame. The *National Directory* is the best of the presently available starting points. It would need to be augmented in two ways. First, facilities without information listings capable of defining whether the housing is congregate housing would have to be called to furnish this information. Clearly noncongregate facilities would be removed. Second, attempts to determine whether any facilities were missed need to be made, through local inquiries to housing network informants.

A sample could then be drawn that would provide a bare minimum amount of descriptive data for the entire sample. Sample facilities then would be visited or telephoned to obtain the third-level and perhaps the second-level data.

Such a project would be very costly. However, until a really major survey of this kind is performed the field will experience the repeated frustrations of having to deal with idiosyncratic site-specific information or small samples of facilities where bias and nonrepresentative distributions are highly likely.

PROCESS RESEARCH

Physical Design Features

The past two decades have produced a heartening rush of collaborations among designers, administrators, social scientists and gerontologists in the task of designing user-friendly environments for older people with different types of needs. The research perspective has characterized this development. The methods employed consist of several different genres. Traditional social-scientific methods with large groups of subjects and formal measurement and analysis have been used in many studies over this period of time. User preference studies have also been ubiquitous, the most sophisticated having been performed by Regnier (1987). The most frequent methodology has consisted of qualitative post-occupancy evaluation, usually in case-study form.

At this point it is difficult to know where design research should go.

There has been little methodological innovation in 20 years. The most useful writing being done now involves collating the findings or opinions of many experts and attempting to find consensus. The most recent example of such consensus research of interest to housing planners is a series of one-sentence design prescriptions grouped under headings such as kitchen, stairs, bathroom, and so on (Prosper, 1990). Such collations are extremely useful, although one must always keep in mind their origin: Informed observations by some writers, plus repetitions of those same observations by many more writers—certainly not the stuff of rigorous science!

This writer is somewhat pessimistic regarding the imminent possibility of notable breakthroughs in testing the outcomes of design alternatives. Two avenues seem the most promising, one on each end of the qualitative-quantitative methodological continuum. On the qualitative side there is room for more formal observation of people actually using their environments. Congregate housing has a greater variety than independent housing of specialized spaces where varied prescribed behaviors occur. The mix of residents with intact and impaired functional capacities also results in a greater range of behaviors being available for observation. Systematic multiple-observer tracking of behaviors such as opening doors, becoming oriented upon entering a building, negotiating the pathway to one's dining room place, choice of seating in public spaces, use of apartment kitchen facilities—the possibilities are limitless—are very likely to improve upon the primarily single-observer sources of design data that one finds in standard writings of this type. Careful representation of differing perspectives is essential for such teams: Architect, administrator, behavior scientist, social worker, for example. A special need is seen for the anthropological perspective, an orientation that is likely to be particularly sensitive to the meaning of the person-environment transactions for the actor and the place of that meaning in the miniature housing culture.

On the quantitative end of the continuum a revival of interest in the ergonomics of aging seems to be occurring, with a recent monograph from the National Research Council (Czaja, 1990) and a special issue of *Human Factors* on this topic now in press. Unlike the situation in environmental psychology, a usable taxonomy of person, environment, and tasks exists for ergonomic research (Gawron et al., 1989), as well as conceptual systems for studying the person-environment interface. Since physical mobility and other activities of daily living are so important in being able to remain in housing (Lawton, in press), rather than an institution, such fine-detailed study of congregate housing tenants interacting with different housing, utensil, and furniture design would seem productive. Extended discussion of research needs in human factors and aging appears in Czaja (1990).

There is doubtless plenty of room for better quantitative evaluations and preference surveys. Too much of such research has begun to repeat earlier investigations, however, to the point where it may be better to wait for some more exciting methods to surface before performing new replications of preferential surveys.

Housing Management

Management as a factor in the efficacy and quality of life in housing environments has been grossly neglected over the years when independent housing flourished. Even less attention has been devoted to the management of congregate housing.

Much of the existing purpose-built congregate housing has been managed by people with some training or background in human-service endeavors. Such administrators are thus likely to be aware of many of the issues in service delivery. The housing they manage entails costs usually well above the costs of subsidized housing. This purpose-built congregate housing can often afford the services of specialists in social work, activities, nursing and other supportive services. In contrast, much of the housing where poor people have aged in place (public housing, primarily) has had very limited management resources from the beginning. Such management often serves mainly a rent-collection and maintenance supervision function, sometimes with a single manager being responsible for several projects.

There is thus considerable ambiguity regarding the role that should be taken by management in dealing with frail elders and their broad social and medical service needs. There is enough diversity in management right now to enable the study of alternative outcomes of congregate housing environments associated with several management types: Management that attempts to incorporate all these roles; management that is mainly physical and financial; and management that allocates these differing functions among specialists in these roles.

Many years ago managerial prototypes of "Marine sergeants" and "bleeding hearts" were described as examples of the widely varying ideologies of management and managers' personalities that might affect tenant well-being (Lawton, 1975). There has still been almost no research addressing the very basic question, "Are there tenant outcomes of any kind that appear to be affected by managerial style?"

The issue of separation of tenants from housing (often involving the move to an institution) has been frequently discussed as a management task but infrequently by empirical research (a notable exception being Sheehan, 1986). Particularly lacking in this area is the ethnographic analysis of the constellation of tenant, family, and management as they deal with increased frailty and the question of remaining versus moving to a higher level of care.

Another set of managerial issues involves management's role in organizing services, a topic to be discussed in the following section.

Congregate Services

The core research issue in congregate housing concerns the service package that defines this housing type. A critical distinction between reasons for offering a service program must be understood from the beginning, the difference between *amenity* services and *supportive* services. Services are used as amenities by people such as those who have always hated food shopping; who think of being served meals as the height of luxury; who seek a socially stimulating environment and view the congregate meals as the vehicle for this goal. The same services may be used as supports by the frail who cannot perform instrumental tasks comfortably on their own.

Aging in place blurs this distinction, of course, with many people choosing services initially as amenities and then coming to require them as their competence declines.

The general research question out of which many specific questions flow is "How does the optimal match between the needs of congregate housing tenants and the services offered affect the overall milieu?"

As noted earlier the *preferences* of older consumers have been studied extensively. Despite such research attention, firm knowledge about what people want is still lacking. For example, as Monk and Kaye (this issue) note, the Malozemoff, Anderson and Rosenbaum (1978) study showed that on-site meals were a very low priority for older residents. This is a very curious finding, in light of the fact that congregate meals form the cornerstone of the genre "congregate housing" and need for such meals constitutes the basic eligibility criterion for CHSP participation. Probing the question regarding consumer demand for meal services requires considerably greater differentiation in constructs and methods than has heretofore been directed to research in this area. It is very likely that economic solvency constitutes the strongest determinant of preference. Full ability to pay for meal service will surely recruit more users to congregate meals for amenity reasons. Poor tenants are correspondingly loath to pay even small amounts for meals. The place of self-efficacy and personal control in such a decision requires study along with SES factors.

The typology of congregate housing residents from the CSHA/NASUA (*Congregate housing*, 1987) report, cited by Monk and Kaye, illustrates this problem well. Diverse motivations for the decision to choose congregate housing need to be understood better before we can design the service programs. The results of such research may inform us whether we should be designing different housing models for services construed as amenities contrasted with those construed as supports. Consumer demand for the CCRC has told us very clearly that few young-old independent older people opt for a service package as complete as that offered by that model. Further exploration may show a relationship between young-old independent people, the amenity model, and fully discretionary meals. Such an environment may be feasible only for the affluent. On the other hand, meals targeted to the frail few in a single housing environment may be possible either in subsidized housing, where the small scale of the congregate meals makes a subsidy for such services necessary; or in high-cost housing where full cost may be borne by the user.

Another congregate meals question requiring study is a more in-depth attempt to determine individual differences in the effect of mandatory meals bundled into a single monthly charge on those who would prefer more control. Outcomes such as dissatisfaction with meals and generalized housing satisfaction are easy to study. It also seems desirable to consider more basic questions such as the effect of cessation of several important instrumental activities (shopping, cooking, cleaning up) on overall independence among people who are both still physically vigorous and who do not wish to take meals with the congregate package.

The thought of "medical services" in congregate housing still evokes negative responses from those who equate any such service with institutional care. There is a very wide range of services that serve health-maintaining purposes short of a full nursing-care environment, however. There is a good reason to feel that the presence of a resident nurse, a physician with regular office hours, or preventive checkup services, contribute to the feeling of security of the resident. Research based on a sample of environments large enough to include some of these major variations ought to inform us about which are most security-inducing and which are unimportant or even actively disliked by the residents. Service-related research that is also relevant to design issues should examine the effects of physical markers of the presence of health services in terms of their obtrusiveness as symbols of illness and a medical milieu.

A very different type of issue in delivery of on-site services is the question of how they should be organized. In earlier research the "patchwork of services" was articulated as the functional equivalent of congregate housing (Lawton, Moss, & Grimes, 1985). The patchwork consists of individual services being delivered by separate agencies, targeted only to those in greatest need, without any central management of the processes of identifying need, prescribing, procuring, and delivering the service.

The patchwork is one of several possible models of service organization, consisting of a service package that "just grew" rather than one that was planned. The traditional congregate housing model is, of course, the most prevalent model. In this model, management is responsible for all services and usually actually delivers the services, with site-employed food service, housekeeping, activities, and other types of staff.

Other models have been proposed, however, often with the thought of reducing the overall costs of the services. The state of Minnesota, for example, has recently decided to offer a single model for existing housing to provide congregate services through a staff care coordinator (Minnesota Board on Aging, 1990). This person is not the administrator but a social-services person placed there by the community agency that sponsors the housing programs. The essence of the care-coordinator model is that costs will be reduced by having a combination of state and local subsidy with mandatory tenant financial participation. Two other models, the Housing Support Services Certificate Program and the Congregate Housing Certificate Program are discussed as future possibilities by Kingsley and Struyk (this issue).

It is clear that the location and affiliation of this coordinator (housing administrator, housing-employed care coordinator, centrally employed care coordinator), the degree of targeting services (one, several, or all services; some or all people), and the recipient of the subsidy if any (the resident, the housing, the service provider) are important parameters whose effects need to be studied.

QUALITY OF LIFE
IN CONGREGATE HOUSING

There has been plenty of research confirming an overall positive effect of congregate housing on quality of life, including many demonstrations of a high level of consumer approval (for example, Lawton, 1976). The type of research now needed concerns changes over longer periods of time in congregate housing environments and the relationships of these changes to the quality of life of older people.

Inevitably questions of this type are closely related to some of the issues already discussed. One focus involves the interaction between targeting of services and the type of resident population as determinants of well-being. Some recommendations from the CHSP evaluation (Sherwood et al., 1985) noted the importance of targeting congregate services to the substantially impaired person if cost savings over institutional care were to be realized (see also Heumann, this issue). Redfoot and Sloan (this issue), on the other hand, suggest that congregate housing is able to serve as a preventive treatment if applied earlier in the trajectory of decline. Thus the range of frailty to which services are to be targeted has both cost and effectiveness implications that deserve further research.

Following the implications of strict targeting at the most vulnerable end of the scale (e.g., three or more daily living impairments) would unquestionably have the negative result predicted by Redfoot and Sloan in a traditional congregate housing environment where all services were provided for all residents. Such an environment would have to be more like assisted living than congregate housing. Services would be easy to apply and certainly cheaper to deliver than the full set of nursing home services. What would the quality of life be, however?

A very researchable issue is the effect of varying mixes of people with differing levels of frailty on overall quality of life of the residents. Strict targeting would result in a very homogeneously frail population. How would the aggregate quality of life of all individuals living there be affected by varying degrees of homogeneity? In this research one would need to examine individual outcomes (i.e., an interaction between an individual's status and overall homogeneity) and aggregate outcomes (quality summed over all residents) to answer this question. It is very important to know how the outcomes associated with a relatively competent person's being in congregate housing differ from those for a relatively impaired person in the same housing.

Such research has been done in elementary and not very satisfactory form (e.g., Lawton, 1976). One problem is the need for enough different housing sites to afford a range of mix of independent and frail persons so the overall effect on individuals may be assessed.

The fact that congregate housing almost always recruits tenants who wish to be served (amenity assistance) and tenants who require service (support) complicates the issue. Having both types of residents seems to be a fact of life. Targeting to the extent recommended by the CHSP evaluation (Sherwood et al., 1985) is probably not even a realistic goal for classic congregate housing where meal services and possibly others have to be supplied to everyone.

Targeting probably is appropriate in the CHSP model where only a proportion of tenants may need any particular service. In this instance the quality of life issue deserving research is the interactions among those receiving services and those not receiving them. Research should ask whether a status differential arises whereby those receiving the services become marked as frail. Do social relationships occur between the frail and the more independent as easily in targeted CHSP-like settings as they do in classic congregate housing where all receive services or in independent housing where the frail are not publicly identified as receivers of service?

Another quality of life issue involves the social relationships among congregate housing residents as the housing environment as a whole ages. Research is clear in showing that physical illness reduces social interaction in normal communities. One would expect that the same tendency would occur as congregate housing ages; that is, tenants become more frail and their social contacts decrease. Is there a process within the congregate context that can counteract such social withdrawal? The idea that congregate meals foster social interaction has never been formally tested, especially the question as to whether people who interact at meals show any generalization to other settings. Explicitly, do congregate tablemates interact away from the meal settings any differently from similarly frail people who do not have the congregate meal setting as a facilitator?

Helping behaviors between frail residents and between frail and independent residents is addressed by Kaye and Monk (this issue). A longitudinal look at the maintenance of earlier relationships as one member of a friendship dyad becomes more frail would be very helpful to both management and to theory in social relationships.

A final area for such research is the relationship between quality of life and the financial costs of different forms of supportive housing. Heumann (this issue) provides a comprehensive view of the costs of congregate housing. Is there any way to turn this kind of research into cost-benefit research? Calculating the monetary value of social and psychological benefits (and costs) is widely recognized as a problem with few promising leads for solutions. One still can hope that measured increments or decrements in social engagement or subjective quality may be estimated. Decision theory has provided novel ways of measuring the subjective value of decrements to quality of life consequent to chronic illness and disability (Kaplan & Bush, 1982; Torrance, 1982). Why not some research asking congregate housing residents to estimate the dollar value of 365 days of the secure feeling that meals and surveillance are available; the value of having a neighbor who notices their presence or absence; the value of feeling that one's domicile is guarded against intrusion; the value of having one friend, two friends, etc.? These suggestions are very primitive at this juncture but that is the way cost-benefit research attempting to combine tangible and intangible goods must begin.

POLICY RESEARCH ON MACROSOCIAL ISSUES

The stream of research by Struyk (1985), Newman and Struyk, 1988) and others (Katsura, Struyk, & Newman, 1988) has used diverse data sets such as the American Housing Survey and the Long Term Care Survey; decennial census data has provided major assistance over the past decade in informing us about national trends. Better information about the housing fate of older people with incomes below the poverty level is required. The American Housing Survey would be greatly improved if the survey schedule could be redesigned to capture more explicitly information about whether the dwelling unit could be characterized as planned housing, whether the occupant has a current housing subsidy (this item is somewhat suspect in quality the way it is asked now), and whether services are delivered. At least on a one-time basis an oversample of older people in planned and/or subsidized housing with an extended section on services and other aging-in-place issues would be very useful for planning purposes.

Extending this wish list even further, this add-on survey could be planned in advance as a 3-year or 5-year longitudinal survey; the AHA is presently longitudinal with respect to the dwelling unit. With proper foresight this feature could be extended as one-time follow-up survey of the subsample of older residents of planned (subsidized housing who had moved to a new dwelling unit.

CONCLUSION

One author's list of research needs constitutes a very defective sample of all such needs. One might hope that this single effort might be followed by a panel with a similar task. It is likely that the federal agency with the most natural vested interest in this topic, the Department of Housing and Urban Development (HUD), will be of no help at all in such an effort. Creative research on congregate housing will cost money and HUD has rarely supported research for the common good. In addition, as stated so eloquently by Redfoot and Sloan (this issue), HUD has good reason to be desperately afraid of research that might question its position against congregate housing or other modes of service delivery.

Therefore one hopes that the National Institute on Aging or the National Institute of Mental Health might see their missions as encompassing the sector of housing research that intersects with frailty and support needs. At the time of this writing, Congressman Roybal has an admirable bill for the increased support of research in the legislative channel (HR4863, 101st Congress). The bill, regrettably, does not do justice to the social and psychological aspects of aging and omits any recognition of the residential aspects of independence and quality of life. Convincing Congress that the area of congregate housing is as relevant to the problems of the frail elderly and the total social structure as is biological aging and Alzheimers disease is an endeavor all housing researchers should join.

REFERENCES

Congregate housing (1987). Washington DC: Council of State Housing Agencies.

Continuing care retirement communities: Analysis and developing trends (1987). Washington DC: American Association of Homes for the Aging.

Continuing care retirement communities: Analysis and developing trends (1989). Washington DC: American Association of Homes for the Aging.

Czaja, S. J. (Ed.). (1990). *Human factors research needs for an aging population*. Washington DC: National Academy of Sciences.

Gawron, V. J., Drury, C. G., Czaja, S. J., & Wilkins, D. M. (1989). A taxonomy of independent variables affecting human performance. *International Journal of Man-Machine Studies, 31*, 643-672.

Kaplan, R. M., & Bush, J. W. (1982). Health-related quality of life measurement for evaluation research and policy analysis. *Health Psychology, 1*, 61-80.

Katsura, H. M., Struyk, R. J., & Newman, S. J. (1988). *Housing for the elderly in 2010: Projections and policy options*. Washington DC: Urban Institute.

Lawton, M. P. (1975). *Planning and managing housing for the elderly*. New York: Wiley-Interscience.

Lawton, M. P. (1976). The relative impact of congregate and traditional housing on elderly tenants. *The Gerontologist, 16*, 237-242.

Lawton, M. P. (1990). Knowledge resources and gaps in housing for the aged. In D. Tillson (Ed.), *Aging in place* (pp.287-309). Glenview IL: Scott Foresman.

Lawton, M. P. (in press). Aging and performance of home tasks. *Human Factors*.

Lawton, M. P., Moss, M., & Grimes, M. (1985). The changing service needs of older tenants in planned housing. *The Gerontologist, 25*, 258-264.

Malozemoff, I. K., Anderson, J. G., & Rosenbaum, L. V. (1978). *Housing for the elderly: Evaluation of the effectiveness of congregate residences*. Boulder CO: Westview Press.

Minnesota Board on Aging (1990). Congregate Housing Services Study. (Duplicated report) St. Paul, Minn.: Minnesota Board on Aging.

Mor, V., Sherwood, S., & Gutkin, C. (1986). A national study of residential care for the aged. *The Gerontologist, 26,* 405-417.

National directory of retirement facilities (1988). Phoenix AZ: Oryx Press.

Newman, S., & Struyk, R. J. (1988). *Housing and supportive services: Federal policy for the frail elderly and chronically mentally ill.* Washington: Urban Institute.

Office of Policy Development and Research (1979). *Housing for the elderly and handicapped.* Washington DC: U.S. Department of Housing and Urban Development.

Prosper, V. (1990). Housing older New Yorkers. 1. Design features. Albany: New York State Office for the Aging.

Regnier, V. (1987). Programming congregate housing: The preferences of upper income elderly. In V. Regnier & J. Pynoos (Eds.). *Housing the aged* (pp.207-226). New York: Elsevier.

Sheehan, N. (1986). Aging of tenants: Termination policy in public senior housing. *The Gerontologist,* 26, 505-509.

Sherwood, S., Morris, J. N., Sherwood, C. C., Morris, S., Bernstein, E., & Gornstein, E. S. (1985). *Evaluation of congregate housing.* Final report, HUD Contract #HC-5373. Boston: Hebrew Rehabilitation Center.

Struyk, R. J. (1985). Future housing assistance policy for the elderly. *The Gerontologist, 25,* 41-46.

Torrance, G. W. (1982). Multiattribute utility theory as a method of measuring social preferences for health states in long-term care. In R. L. Kane & R. A. Kane (Eds.). *Values and long-term care* (pp.127-156). Lexington MA: Lexington Books.

Index